ADVANCED PRACTICE
NURSING

CONTEXTS OF CARE

EDITED BY:

LYNETTE HAMLIN, PHD, RN, CNM, FACNM

President
KAM Learning, LLC
Inman, South Carolina

Associate Dean of Nursing
Saint Joseph's College
Standish, Maine

JONES & BARTLETT
LEARNING

World Headquarters
Jones & Bartlett Learning
5 Wall Street
Burlington, MA 01803
978-443-5000
info@jblearning.com
www.jblearning.com

Jones & Bartlett Learning books and products are available through most bookstores and online booksellers. To contact Jones & Bartlett Learning directly, call 800-832-0034, fax 978-443-8000, or visit our website, www.jblearning.com.

Substantial discounts on bulk quantities of Jones & Bartlett Learning publications are available to corporations, professional associations, and other qualified organizations. For details and specific discount information, contact the special sales department at Jones & Bartlett Learning via the above contact information or send an email to specialsales@jblearning.com.

The content, statements, views, and opinions herein are the sole expression of the respective authors and not that of Jones & Bartlett Learning, LLC. Reference herein to any specific commercial product, process, or service by trade name, trademark, manufacturer, or otherwise does not constitute or imply its endorsement or recommendation by Jones & Bartlett Learning, LLC and such reference shall not be used for advertising or product endorsement purposes. All trademarks displayed are the trademarks of the parties noted herein. *Advanced Practice Nursing: Contexts of Care* is an independent publication and has not been authorized, sponsored, or otherwise approved by the owners of the trademarks or service marks referenced in this product.

There may be images in this book that feature models; these models do not necessarily endorse, represent, or participate in the activities represented in the images. Any screenshots in this product are for educational and instructive purposes only. Any individuals and scenarios featured in the case studies throughout this product may be real or fictitious, but are used for instructional purposes only.

The authors, editor, and publisher have made every effort to provide accurate information. However, they are not responsible for errors, omissions, or for any outcomes related to the use of the contents of this book and take no responsibility for the use of the products and procedures described. Treatments and side effects described in this book may not be applicable to all people; likewise, some people may require a dose or experience a side effect that is not described herein. Drugs and medical devices are discussed that may have limited availability controlled by the Food and Drug Administration (FDA) for use only in a research study or clinical trial. Research, clinical practice, and government regulations often change the accepted standard in this field. When consideration is being given to use of any drug in the clinical setting, the health care provider or reader is responsible for determining FDA status of the drug, reading the package insert, and reviewing prescribing information for the most up-to-date recommendations on dose, precautions, and contraindications, and determining the appropriate usage for the product. This is especially important in the case of drugs that are new or seldom used.

Production Credits

Executive Publisher: William Brottmiller
Executive Editor: Amanda Martin
Associate Managing Editor: Sara Bempkins
Production Manager: Carolyn Rogers Pershouse
Production Editor: Sarah Bayle
Senior Marketing Manager: Jennifer Stiles
VP, Manufacturing and Inventory Control:
  Therese Connell
Composition: diacriTech
Cover Design: Kristin E. Parker
Manager of Photo Research, Rights & Permissions:
  Lauren Miller
Cover Image: © LeksusTuss/ShutterStock, Inc.
Printing and Binding: Edwards Brothers Malloy
Cover Printing: Edwards Brothers Malloy

Library of Congress Cataloging-in-Publication Data
Advanced practice nursing (Hamlin)
Advanced practice nursing : contexts of care / [edited by] Lynette Hamlin.
    p. ; cm.
Includes bibliographical references and index.
ISBN 978-1-284-04702-8
I. Hamlin, Lynette, editor. II. Title.
[DNLM: 1. Advanced Practice Nursing—methods—United States—Case Reports.
2. Advanced Practice Nursing—standards—United States—Case Reports. WY 128]
RT51
610.73—dc23
                                                                    2014009969
6048

Printed in the United States of America
18 17 16 15 14   10 9 8 7 6 5 4 3 2 1

Dedication

To my three daughters, Kaitlyn DeMarsico,
Alyssa Ament, and Mallory Ament,
for your patience and support in all my endeavors.

Contents

Chapter 7   Health Policy and Advocacy: Practice to the Full Extent

Mary Virden, RN, MSEd

Chapter 8   Patient Safety: Congressional Action

Angela S. Mattie, JD, MPH

Chapter 12 The Clinical Nurse Leader   **261**

Pamela Abraham, MSN, RN, CNL, Catherine Edmonds,
MSN, RN, CNL, Jennifer Kareivis, MSN, RN, CNL,
and Marianne Sweeney, MSN, RN, CNL

Chapter 13 Disaster Preparedness   **283**

Dottie Bringle, RN, BSN, MSHSA, COO/CNO,
Mercy-Joplin Hospital

Chapter 14 Power in the Healthcare Relationship   **299**

Judith B. Krauss, RN, MSN, FAAN

Acknowledgments

This work is truly the concept of Donna Diers. She designed the course, "Contexts of Care," for the graduate students at Yale School of Nursing. An inspirational woman with great vision, Donna mentored many in their careers, including me. Many thanks also go to Judith Krauss and Sally Cohen, who through their work in the YSN Center for Health Policy and Ethics have expanded the original work of "Contexts of Care" and broadened the perspectives of advanced practice nursing students. This work would not be possible without the efforts and support of many.

© Leksustuss/ShutterStock, Inc

Preface

This book is written for nursing students and faculty to use as health policy cases worthy of discussion, debate, and dissection. There are many excellent texts about the history of U.S. health policy and current health policy trends; these cases have been written to apply to health policy issues. The concept belongs to Donna Diers; she invited me to join her course as a member of her teaching team. I feel strongly that these concepts, and these stories, are important to share and use as learning moments.

About the Author

Lynette Hamlin, PhD, RN, CNM, FACNM, received her Bachelor of Science in Nursing and Master of Science in Nursing degrees from Loyola University of Chicago, her post-master's certificate in nurse-midwifery from the University of Illinois, and her doctorate in nursing, with a minor in public administration, from the University of Wisconsin–Milwaukee. Dr. Hamlin has held academic leadership positions at Yale University School of Nursing, University of New Hampshire, and University of South Carolina Upstate. She has extensive experience as both a nursing and midwifery educator and a clinician. She is a fellow in the American College of Nurse-Midwives, a participant in the U.S. Department of Health and Human Services 2003 Primary Health Care Policy Fellowship, and a recipient of the coveted Kitty Ernst Award.

Reviewers

Marguerite Ambrose, PhD, ACNS, BC
Associate Professor
Immaculata University
Immaculata, Pennsylvania

Pamela Bjorklund, PhD, APRN, CNS, PMHNP-BC
Associate Professor
Department of Graduate Nursing
The College of St. Scholastica
Duluth, Minnesota

Kelly L. Fisher, PhD, RN
Dean and Associate Professor in Nursing
Endicott College
Beverly, Massachusetts

Monica Flowers, FNP-BC, DNP
Clinical Assistant Professor
Florida International University
Miami, Florida

Janis Waite Hayden, RN, MSN, EdD
Professor
Saint Francis Medical Center College of Nursing
Peoria, Illinois

Layna Himmelberg, EdD, RN, CNE
Associate Professor
Clarkson College
Omaha, Nebraska

Theresa A. Hoadley, PhD, RN, MS, BSN
Associate Professor, Lead Faculty
Saint Francis Medical Center College of Nursing
Peoria, Illinois

Kelly A. Kuhns, PhD, RN
Assistant Professor
Millersville University
Millersville, Pennsylvania

Connie Lapadat, MSN-FNP-C
Assistant Professor
American Public College
University of Northern British Columbia
Vancouver, Canada

Carolyn T. LePage, PhD, ARNP-C
Family Nurse Practitioner
Barry University College of Health Sciences
Miami Shores, Florida

Daniel J. Little, PhD, MBA, MSN, ARNP, ACNP, FNP-BC
Assistant Clinical Professor of Nursing, Foreign Educated Physicians
    Program
Florida International University
Nicole Werthheim College of Nursing and Health Science
Biscayne Bay Campus
North Miami, Florida

Angela Stone Schmidt, PhD, MNSc, RNP, RN
Associate Dean, Director of Graduate Programs
College of Nursing & Health Professions
Arkansas State University
Jonesboro, Arkansas

Patricia A. Senk, PhD
Assistant Professor
The College of St. Scholastica
Duluth, Minnesota

Carole A. Shea, PhD, RN, FAAN
Professor Emerita
California State University, Dominguez Hills
Carson, California

Terri Shumway, MSN, FNP-BC
Assistant Professor, Lead Faculty FNP Program
Saint Francis Medical Center College of Nursing
Peoria, Illinois

Contributors

Pamela Abraham, MSN, RN, CNL
Hunterdon Medical Center
Flemington, New Jersey

B. J. Bockenhauer, MSN, APRN, PMH-CNS-BC
Private Practice
Concord, New Hampshire

Dottie Bringle, RN, BSN, MSHSA
Chief Operating Officer/Chief Nursing Officer
St. John's Regional Medical Center
Joplin, Missouri

Kelly Cummings, RN
New Hampshire Hospital
Concord, New Hampshire

Catherine Edmonds, MSN, RN, CNL
Hunterdon Medical Center
Flemington, New Jersey

Jean Johnson, PhD, RN, FAAN
Dean and Professor
The George Washington University School of Nursing
Washington, D.C.

Jennifer Kareivis, MSN, RN, CNL
Hunterdon Medical Center
Flemington, New Jersey

Kathleen Kimmel, RN, BSN, MHA, FHIMSS
Chief Nursing Officer
MedeAnalytics
Emeryville, California

Judith Krauss, MSN, RN, FAAN
Professor, Yale University School of Nursing
Master, Silliman College
New Haven, Connecticut

Linda Searle Leach, PhD, RN, NEA-BC, CNL
Assistant Professor
UCLA School of Nursing
UCLA Health System Patient Safety Institute
Los Angeles, California

Angela Mattie, JD, MPH
Associate Professor of Management
Chair, Health Care Management & Organizational Leadership
Quinnipiac University
Hamden, Connecticut

Christine Pintz, PhD, MSN
Associate Professor
Director, DNP Program
The George Washington University School of Nursing
Washington, D.C.

Lynn Price, JD, MS, MPH, MSN
Professor of Nursing
Director, Graduate Nursing
Quinnipiac University
Hamden, Connecticut

Robin Raiford, RN-BC, CPHIMS, FHIMSS
Research Director
Advisory Board Company
Washington, D.C.

Susan Reeves, EdD
Associate Academic Dean for Dartmouth-Hitchcock Partnership
    Program
The Gladys A. Burrows Distinguished Professor of Nursing Chair,
Nursing Public Health
Colby-Sawyer College
New London, New Hampshire

Marianne Sweeney, MSN, RN, CNL
Hunterdon Medical Center
Flemington, New Jersey

Julie Jacobson Vann, PhD, MS, RN
Senior Researcher, Health Program
American Institutes for Research
Washington, D.C.

Mary D. Virden, MSE, RN
Clinical Assistant Professor
School of Nursing Administrator, Silver City Health Center
Director, Clinical Services, KU HealthPartners, Inc.
The University of Kansas Medical Center
Kansas City, Kansas

CHAPTER 1

Contexts of Care

Lynette Hamlin, PhD, RN, CNM, FACNM

The context of whom we provide care to matters. One might argue that the context of how, where, when, and why we provide care matters even more. Considering context is of paramount importance because the delivery of care first is influenced at the microsystem level and subsequently exerts an effect on the larger delivery system. To be complete, this discussion must also recognize that the macro system has an effect that filters to the microsystem. The sum of these forces and complexities manifests in our patient outcomes (Nelson, Batalden, & Godfrey, 2007) and, ultimately, perpetuates health policy as well as dictates future policy.

In this text, the complexities of our healthcare system and the forces that shape policy are illustrated through examples of personal stories that describe actual events. The stories capture the pressures and realities of wading through a complex healthcare system in the efforts to provide care and support professional nursing (Diers, 2002). The policies and regulations of our ever-changing healthcare system affect our ability to provide safe care within our individual ethical perspectives. And when we try to function in our organizational microsystems, encompassed by macro system organizational culture, we are forced to consider the influence of those policies on our care. These stories are written so that you must uncover the incomplete or sometimes contradictory information that is available and analyze the "what ifs." The authors ask what you would do if you were faced with these circumstances. What data would you need to collect? Who is the keeper of the data, or do the data even exist? What resources would you need? Who can provide those resources? How will you interface with the players? Are all of the necessary players at the table, and if not, how will you get them there? What would you like to see as the end result? Are there any adverse outcomes you would like to avoid, and if so, what quality improvement and/or safety initiatives can you implement to avoid them? There are no right or wrong answers.

In *Contexts of Care* you are asked to critically analyze the stories. The stories come with discussion questions. You are free to use them to guide your analysis or not. You are challenged to apply new theories and knowledge to events in a manner that generates solutions. As practitioners, we tend to focus on the how-to of providing competent care and seek a road map that includes detailed position descriptions for our role. Yet as advanced practice nurses, we cannot separate the practice issues from the policy issues. Everything we do on a daily basis is underpinned by current healthcare policy.

These stories provide you with an insider's view of the context in which care is provided (Diers, 2002). From this view, you can summarize the various pressures and considerations that the story's narrator faced. If you read between the lines, you will gain a better understanding of the importance of context. Through context we find order in the world and a sharpened perspective on reality, which in turn provide a backdrop for further development and refinement of our practice.

One note of caution: These stories take place at various times along the timeline of health care. The dates of the cases may be important to the understanding what options were available to the actors. Remember that it is not fair to criticize an institution, organization, or individual for not playing by rules that weren't invented yet (Diers, 2002). Even if some cases seem "old," they were chosen purposefully to represent issues that, although the facts or regulations or politics may have changed, remain current (Diers, 2002).

The stories are meant to be discussed in groups—analyzed, debated, negotiated, strategized, and more. You are challenged to collaborate with others to resolve the issues presented in the stories, present alternative actions not taken by the actors in the stories, generate further questions, and provide evidence to support your conclusions. Health policy is made, changed, and implemented on several levels. These stories are a cross-match of policy issues that occur on the individual provider level, the organizational level, and the local, regional, and national levels. Analyzing and evaluating stories that occur in the context of time and politics are ideal ways to strategize and break apart options, solutions, and outcomes (Diers, Gustafson, Mahrenholz, & Price, 2002). Will you negotiate, argue, or attempt to convince your colleagues of your conclusions? The contexts of these stories serve as a reminder that health policy also has a context. How would these stories change, or not, in the context of today's healthcare environment?

How to Use This Text

For learning to occur with case method teaching, the learner must accept responsibility for learning and then share that learning with colleagues. Case method teaching is not just about reading a story and providing solutions derived from your personal experiences or assumptions. As with any endeavor, a thorough analysis involves gathering data, synthesizing data, and then applying data. The references and additional resources sections can be used as background or to tease out the context of the story. You will have to seek out additional information and evidence through readings or references to help you build the competency necessary to improve the health outcomes of your clients and the quality of your healthcare delivery system.

The backdrop for these stories is professional reports and standards for health care and nursing: the Institute of Medicine (IOM) reports (IOM, 1999, 2003a, 2003b, 2010), the Quality and Safety Education for Nurses (QSEN) graduate competencies (QSEN Institute, n.d.), and the Essentials of Master's Education in Nursing (American Association of Colleges of Nursing, 2011). The stories are organized around the following themes: scope of practice, organizational and systems leadership, finance and regulatory environments, interprofessional collaboration, quality improvement and safety, professional ethics, evidence-based practice, clinical prevention and population health, and informatics.

Master's-educated healthcare professionals must be prepared as leaders with the ability to act critically within complex and ever-changing healthcare systems. We must advocate for our consumers, ourselves, and our profession to shape the future of our healthcare delivery system. We need to hold ourselves accountable for the quality of care delivered, the manner of care delivered, and the cost of care delivered.

You will find three basic chapter formats: in some chapters, the author has written text to introduce the subject matter and then concludes the chapter with a series of illustrative case studies; in other chapters, the author covers multiple subtopics, inserting illustrative case studies related to each topic throughout; and in the final format, the chapter is comprised of a single comprehensive case study. All chapters have multiple discussion questions inserted throughout to help you develop your thoughts in the following areas:

- Identify the problem and define the issue.
- Identify the stakeholders.
- Identify the risks and benefits to the stakeholders.
- Analyze the impact of the issue on the macro system, whether it is the organization or the larger healthcare system.
- Assemble your evidence—information/data that affect your beliefs about the case.
- Evaluate potential solutions to the issues.
- Construct a plan of action.
- Develop an analysis of potential outcomes.
- Evaluate the policy implications of your plan.

You can choose a format to present your analysis. Examples of the ways other learners have presented their analysis are as follows:

- A memo to an appropriate agency official
- A briefing paper to a senator
- A letter to the editor written from a particular point of view (e.g., CEO's, a regulatory agency's, an affected party's)

Nursing occurs within a context that inevitably influences both practice and policy. On the journey you experience through these stories, you will begin to understand how nursing's history has shaped trends and issues into contemporary practice and how nursing has come to value experience as data. It is my hope that you realize that how you choose to integrate your understandings into your own practice may ultimately determine nursing's future, as well as your own.

References

American Association of Colleges of Nursing. (2011). *The essentials of master's education in nursing.* Washington, DC: Author.

Diers, D. (2002). *Contexts of care syllabus.* New Haven, CT: Yale University School of Nursing.

Diers, D., Gustafson, E., Mahrenholz, D., & Price, L. (2002). *Case method learning, Contexts of care course presentation.* New Haven, CT: Yale University School of Nursing.

Institute of Medicine. (1999). *To err is human: Building a safer health system.* Washington, DC: Author.

Institute of Medicine. (2003a). *Health professions education: A bridge to quality.* Washington, DC: Author.

Institute of Medicine. (2003b). *Keeping patients safe: Transforming the work environment of nurses.* Washington, DC: Author.

Institute of Medicine. (2010). *The future of nursing: Leading change, advancing health.* Washington, DC: Author.

Nelson, E. C., Batalden, P. B., & Godfrey, M. M. (2007). *Quality by design: A clinical microsystems approach.* San Francisco, CA: Jossey-Bass.

QSEN Institute. (n.d.). Graduate KSAs. Retrieved from http://qsen.org/competencies/graduate-ksas/

CHAPTER 2

Advanced Practice Nursing and Governance

Susan A. Reeves, EdD, RN

© LeksusTuss/ShutterStock, Inc.

Learning Objectives

At the completion of this chapter, you will be able to:

1. Explain the significance of organizational structure to the role and power base of the APRN.
2. Analyze fiscal pressures placed on clinicians in relation to the concept of productivity.
3. Envision a professional practice environment in which an APRN is optimally deployed and valued as an integral and essential member of the healthcare team.
4. Explore key organizational relationships that are essential when planning significant change.
5. Examine opportunities for meaningful partnerships with chief nursing officers of healthcare organizations.

In this case, environmental and fiscal pressures converge to threaten the job security of more than 200 Advanced Practice Registered Nurses (APRNs) within a large, multispecialty physician group practice at a rural academic medical center. A particular group of APRNs explores new organizational relationships and resources in an attempt to respond proactively to the crisis. The APRNs must confront personal biases and deep-seated organizational culture biases to make the changes in their model of care delivery that will ensure this ongoing role in patient care. Establishing a linkage with a pivotal nursing leader proves to be the key to the group's success.

BOX 2-1: *Core Dimensions of Professional Governance Models*

Professional control over practice

Organizational influence of professionals over resources that support practice

Organizational recognition of professional control and influence

Facilitating structures for participation in decision making

Liaison between professional and administrative groups for access to information

Alignment of organizational and professional goals and negotiation of conflict

Source: Data from Hess, R. G. (1998). Measuring nursing governance. *Nursing Research, 47*(1), 35–42.

Part I: Background

Valley Medical Center (VMC) is a rural academic institution with a 500-bed inpatient hospital (full service) and a large, multispecialty physician group practice with more than 400 physicians. The nursing division of the hospital is well known for its early adoption in the late 1970s of clinical nurse specialist practice as well as its innovation with professional governance models for staff nurses.

As the role and specialty practice of the APRN began to expand in the 1990s, the number of advanced practice nurses (APNs) grew rapidly at VMC. Today there are more than 200 APNs employed by the medical group practice, including Certified

Registered Nurse Anesthetists (CRNAs), Neonatal Nurse Practitioners (NNPs), Certified Nurse–Midwives (CNMs), clinical care APRNs, and a multitude of primary and tertiary care APRNs.

Because the APN role at VMC emerged within the physician group practice (the organization that provided the APNs with credentialing and privileging benefits and supervision), very little interface with the hospital-based division of nursing was established. A relationship with the chief nursing officer (CNO) of the medical center is lacking. (Also note that a centralized nursing organization for the multitude of practices and clinics in the medical group practice is also absent.)

For years, this separatist model of nursing practice administration operated quite well. For those rare times when a unified nursing organization across VMC was called for (such as during an accreditation visit by the Joint Commission and, later, when the organization was applying for Magnet designation by the American Nurses Credentialing Center), "box and line" organization charts were created that demonstrated "dotted line" relationships between the advanced practice nurses in the group practices and the CNO of the medical center. The arms-length relationship was effective from an operating standpoint and so was expanded, codified, and enculturated for years.

DISCUSSION QUESTIONS

1. Using a box and line chart, diagram the reporting relationships for the APRNs in your operating unit.

2. Where is professional practice for an advanced practice nurse in your organization discussed? How are policies for APRN practice developed and updated?

3. Does an individual with intimate knowledge of APRN practice and regulation within the state oversee the privileging of APRNs in your organization?

Part II: Economic Realities of the 2000s Set In

As the number of APNs in the VMC organization grew, so did the diversity of roles. With the implementation of the 2002 Graduate Medical Education 80-hour work week rule for resident physicians, numerous APNs were recruited by the specialty physicians group to provide essential coverage for the inpatient services, critical care areas, and emergency department. Each specialty physician group sought to credential and privilege the APNs, known as "resident extenders," in the group's own specific specialty skills and procedures.

In the outpatient clinics, APNs further extended physician practice in specialty areas by carrying full outpatient client responsibilities. Such activities provided time and coverage for physicians to engage in research and education of medical residents. The physician service chief functioned as the leader for all physicians, residents, and APNs within a specialty area. Few, if any, relationships among APNs across the organization existed.

As the mid-2000s arrived, significant reductions in funding for physician services began to erode the bottom line of the nation's physician organizations. Academic medical centers

---

BOX 2-2: *Productivity = Value / Time*

There are two ways to increase productivity:

1. Increase the value created.
2. Decrease the time required to create that value.

For a concise discussion of productivity, see Steve Pavlina's blog post at www.stevepavlina.com/blog/2005/10/what-is-productivity/.

Clinical productivity is commonly measured in the outpatient setting using relative value units (RVUs). RVUs are standardized, weighted measures that comprise estimates of clinician work (time and intensity of service), practice expense, and malpractice expense. A helpful primer on RVUs as a measure of productivity is from the National Health Policy Forum at www.nhpf.org/library/the-basics/basics_rvus_02-12-09.pdf.

Consider also: Kleinpell, R. M. (2013). *Outcomes assessment in advanced practice nursing* (3rd ed.). New York, NY: Springer.

(AMCs), often serving as a region's healthcare safety net for the underserved and uninsured, were particularly hard hit financially.

VMC's board of trustees appropriately began to exert pressure on the management staff to enhance physician productivity in all areas of practice. Because VMC was rurally sited, essentially no new markets were waiting to be developed to provide new patients for VMC. With no new additional sources of patient revenue available to enhance productivity, a reduction in clinician staff would become inevitable.

As the physician service chiefs came to terms with the magnitude of practice change required to achieve new relative value unit (RVU) and visit volume targets, it was increasingly clear that all clinician roles would be closely examined, realigned, and, if necessary, eliminated. Many of the VMC APNs grew concerned about how they would fare in this dynamic environment; several, particularly those practicing as a solo APN in a medical specialty group, felt especially vulnerable.

DISCUSSION QUESTIONS

1. Why did the pressure to increase physician productivity cause the APNs to grow concerned?

2. Other than RVUs, what other measures might be useful to demonstrate contributions of the APN to patient care?

3. What proactive communication or meeting might the APNs have considered as the service chiefs embarked on making changes in the various areas?

Part III: A Path Forward

The Cancer Center at VMC employed one of the largest cohorts of APNs in the physician group practices. When the service chiefs began to plan meetings with their clinician groups to discuss impending changes in the work of the members, Elaine, the longest-tenured, informal leader of the APN group, called an after-hours meeting of the APNs. The purpose of this meeting, she said, was to share information and brainstorm potential responses to the job security threat the APNs were experiencing.

As the meeting progressed, it became clear that, even within the operating unit of the Cancer Center, wide variation existed in the roles of the APNs. Some saw patients with their physician colleagues; others had more independent practices and had individual appointments with patients. In some practices (subspecialty disease groupings such as breast cancer specialists, gastrointestinal cancer specialists, etc.), APNs billed for visits; in others, no bill was issued. Some APNs covered the inpatient services, and others were on call. Some covered telephone triage, and others, the chemotherapy infusion center. In one area, radiation oncology, the APNs' role was to intervene with patients requiring symptom management.

An interesting commonality among the APNs was their weekly "academic day" when they could develop their own scholarship or research program. This opportunity was modeled on their physician counterparts' method of career advancement, which, unlike the APNs', was linked to research productivity. On this day, the APNs participated in many non-patient-care activities that provided personal and professional satisfaction. Many were leaders in professional societies and research cooperative groups, while others regularly contributed scholarly work to specialty journals. The APNs were especially concerned about losing their "academic day" in the new environment.

Elaine, an APN in the oncology service, began to see that the group needed help thinking through options that could be presented to the service chiefs—options that could continue to meet the goals of providing high-quality cancer care while enhancing clinical productivity (revenue). She suggested reaching out to VMC's new chief nursing officer, Anne Butler. Anne, though virtually unknown to the APN group, was a strong nursing advocate and proponent of professional governance models for staff nurses. Elaine was hopeful that Anne might have some guidance for the oncology APN group.

DISCUSSION QUESTIONS

1. Of the various practice models in which the oncology APNs were engaged, which increased their vulnerability during efforts to enhance productivity? Why?

2. How is the APNs' academic day both an opportunity and a threat in the new environment?

3. Are there models that quantify productivity in research settings? Education settings? How might the APNs characterize the value of their collective academic and professional activity outputs in a way that would be meaningful and beneficial to VMC? The Cancer Center?

Part IV: Linking with the Nursing Division: One Step Forward, Two Steps Back?

The day following the APN meeting, as Elaine was packing up after a long day in the lung cancer clinic, three of her APN colleagues appeared in her doorway and asked to talk more about Elaine's plan to contact the CNO for help with their situation.

"Do you really think it's a good idea to try and get support from the nursing division?" asked one of the APNs. A second said, "We've worked so hard to become meaningful participants in the physician group practice that to go back and align with nursing seems like a step backward." The third indicated, "I doubt the CNO knows anything about advanced practice nursing!"

The first speaker went on, "Don't you think it might make more sense to try and establish our own APN model within the physician practice and have a leader who has the same status as the service chiefs with a seat at their decision-making table? We just aren't nurses like those in the nursing division anymore. We're different."

Elaine understood the sentiments her colleagues expressed. But she also was very concerned about the level of tension and pressure in the physician group at the moment. Even though the physicians were their close, working colleagues, she knew that many physician-only meetings were occurring and no one seemed to be appreciating the APNs as co-equal peers in these meetings. In fact, the APNs were not even invited to contribute ideas about the productivity goals and how to restructure the practices to achieve them.

Elaine said to her peers, "I understand your points, but honestly, this train has left the station and we aren't on it. I'm banking on the fact that not only will Anne be an advocate for us but that she'll also have some ideas for us. I'll arrange a time to go and talk with her, and then maybe have her come to a meeting with all of us. Give me few days and then we can talk again."

DISCUSSION QUESTIONS

1. What possible issues underlie the APNs' concerns about alignment with the nursing division?

2. What could have motivated the APN's comment that to align with the nursing division is a "step backward"?

3. As Elaine makes preparations to meet with Anne, what might be the speaking points she can plan to cover? Questions she might ask?

4. What was your reaction to the comment, "We just aren't like the nurses in the nursing division anymore"? How would you respond to the comment if someone said this to you?

Part V: Anne Butler, Chief Nursing Officer

Anne, chief nursing officer, had arrived at VMC 10 months ago. Previously a successful CNO at a large metropolitan teaching hospital for 15 years, she made the move in hopes of improving her lifestyle. The chance to work in an academic medical center in a rural setting fit the bill perfectly.

Since her arrival at VMC, Anne worked closely with the nurses in the hospital nursing division to establish a professional governance model. The model included quality and safety improvement programs, a clinical and administrative policy committee, as well as clinical excellence recognition and career advancement programs. The satisfaction measures for the nurses in the division were at an all-time high, and there was planning under way to apply for Magnet recognition. The physician group practice leaders were both enthusiastic and supportive of Anne's goals for nursing because they could easily perceive the benefits to the entire organization of a high-performing nursing division.

Anne was intrigued by Elaine's request for a meeting. Early on, Anne had tried to establish some kind of relationship with the APNs in the group practice but had found it difficult to know where to connect, given the vast decentralization of the APNs within the group. It seemed that as she learned about one APN's roles, they were nothing like the next APN's.

Anne experienced a bit of low-level anxiety about the vast APN cohort in the group practice because, at least on the paper organizational chart, she had a "dotted line" relationship for the purpose of overall nursing practice supervision. She knew the former CNO had no relationship with the APNs. In fact, when Anne started at VMC, she had been told that she "didn't have to worry about the APNs in the group practice because they were well supervised by the service chiefs."

At any rate, Anne was pleased by Elaine's overture and looked forward to their scheduled meeting. Although she had no illusions that Elaine represented all of the APNs in the group practice, she knew that the oncology APNs were among the largest clusters of APNs at VMC. If she could make some inroads with the oncology group, it could be a great place to begin to exert some influence and lead the rest of the APNs.

DISCUSSION QUESTIONS

1. What are common elements of professional governance models in nursing? Might a professional governance model for the APNs be a potential avenue to address the present challenges? What would be the pros and cons of developing such a model? Where might one begin?

2. Could the APNs explore other potential forms of collective action? What are the strengths and weaknesses of such models?

3. What useful data should Anne gather to inform her meeting with Elaine?

Part VI: Meeting with Anne

Elaine related to her oncology APN colleagues that the meeting with Anne went exceptionally well. Anne understood the challenges (financial, operational, and professional) that the physician group was experiencing and knew, specifically, about the nitty-gritty details of the oncology practices. Anne agreed that the job security concerns the oncology APN group perceived were real and that a bold plan to address both the organization's and the APNs' needs was in order.

Anne soon met with the entire oncology APN group and began to help them develop a professional practice model. Anne worked with the physician director of the Cancer Center to pave the way for the work. She assured the director that any model developed would positively address the productivity concerns. The director then communicated Anne's plans to the various service chiefs, who, if truth be told, were relieved that their APN colleagues were receiving help and support because, other than eliminating positions, they were not sure what else to do.

In the first meeting with the oncology APN group, Anne made a very strategic move by acknowledging potential concerns about linking with the nursing division. She acknowledged that the APN role was different from the roles in the nursing division. However, she stressed that the advanced practice nursing role was, after all, still a nursing role. Further, she talked about sources of power in organizations and suggested that expecting the physician group to advocate equally for APNs in the current climate was unlikely—not because the APNs were not individually valued as colleagues, but because the physician group practice would first ensure the viability of the physician positions in the group before concerning itself with the "midlevel provider" staff.

Anne knowledgeably discussed the contributions APNs could make in the oncology practice. She also highlighted areas of unmet patient need that could represent as yet untapped sources of volume (revenue) that the APNs were uniquely qualified to manage (symptom management, emergent care or triage, ongoing assessments for patients receiving chemotherapy or radiation treatments, palliative care, pain management, advance directive counseling, support groups, inpatient consultation, etc.).

In subsequent meetings, Anne helped the group conceive of a group practice model that was linked not only to their services but also to the nursing division at large. As the APNs developed their model, a more consistent role and set of expectations for the APNs emerged that resulted in very high levels of performance and satisfaction.

Anne continued to keep the Cancer Center director abreast of the work and relied on the Cancer Center director to help with removing obstacles to the changes the APNs were making. Within 6 months, the oncology APNs made a presentation to the Cancer Center physician staff to announce this new practice model as well as the expected "contribution to financial margin" the model implementation would realize. No reductions in APN staff were recommended. The work of the Cancer Center APNs was cited by the leaders of the physician group practice as proactive, innovative, and responsive to the challenges VMC faced. The leaders encouraged other specialty sections in the practices to disseminate the model more widely in the organization.

Part VII: Epilogue

Anne worked tirelessly over the next several years to encourage and invite APN participation in the professional governance nursing division of VMC. As the APNs began to actively and broadly participate in practice and administrative work, the collective quality and reputation of nursing at VMC grew by leaps and bounds. Magnet status was awarded to VMC 3 years after Anne's tenure began. Five years later, Anne, who until that time was the only voting nurse member of the VMC internal governing body, was thrilled to learn that staff nurse and advanced practice nursing chairs of the nursing division's Professional Governance Model would be invited to join her as additional voting members.

BOX 2-3: *Contributions APNs Can Make in Magnet-Designed Nursing Organizations*

Developer of clinical expertise in nursing staff

Contributor to knowledge development and leader in clinical and system improvement processes

Role model for

Teaching excellence

Competence in interprofessional collaboration and teamwork

Professional autonomy in practice

Evaluator of care quality using data and analytic techniques

Employer of timely consultation and judicious utilization of resources

Interpreter of available evidence for use in nursing practice

Mentor, coach, and collegial supporter for all nursing staff

DISCUSSION QUESTIONS

1. What strategies did Anne employ early in her relationship with the oncology APNs?

2. Why was Anne's relationship with the director of the Cancer Center so crucial in the process?

3. How would Anne's approach need to have changed when she worked with specialty sections that had only one APN?

4. What skills and knowledge did the APN group likely need during the time that they developed their professional practice model? What resources may have been beneficial in the process, and where might they be located?

5. How would one evaluate the success of the new APN practice model? What measures would be crucial in an evaluation?

Reference

Hess, R. G. (1998). Measuring nursing governance. *Nursing Research, 47*(1), 35–42.

Additional Resources

American Nurses Credentialing Center. (n.d.). Announcing a new model for ANCC's Magnet Recognition Program. Retrieved from http://www.nursecredentialing.org/MagnetModel.aspx

Hamric, A., Spross, J., & Hanson, C. (2009). *Advanced nursing practice: An integrative approach.* St. Louis, MO: Elsevier Saunders.

Ives Erickson, J., Jones, D., & Ditomassi, M. (2013). *Fostering nurse led care: Professional practice for the bedside leader from Massachusetts General Hospital.* Indianapolis, IN: Sigma Theta Tau International.

Kleinpell, R. M. (2013). *Outcomes assessment in advanced practice nursing* (3rd ed.). New York, NY: Springer.

CHAPTER 3

Advanced Practice and Prescriptive Authority

Lynn Price, JD, MSN, MPH

Learning Objectives

At the completion of this chapter, you will be able to:

1. Identify formal and informal barriers that restrict scope of APN practice.
2. Outline the steps from bill to law.
3. Differentiate between statutes and regulations.
4. Strategize to identify allies and partners for nursing.
5. Examine the source and rationale for barriers to advanced practice.
6. Propose action plans to remove barriers to advanced practice nursing.

Background

Under the U.S. Constitution, the responsibility to safeguard public health is left to each state to regulate. And states, of course, differ in how they approach public safety. For instance, some states require motorcyclists to wear helmets; others do not. State laws regarding prescriptive authority for advanced practice nurses (APNs) vary widely, as does the structure under which APNs may prescribe. In fact, there are tremendous differences among the states in how and what APNs may prescribe.

Whereas the education, certification, and skills required to practice as an APN do not differ markedly from state to state, the ability to practice fully depends absolutely on where an APN decides to practice. As you read this case, note the formal and informal barriers that prohibit full APN prescriptive authority and other practice.

The beginnings of advanced practice nursing can best be traced to the introduction of nurse midwifery in the United States in 1925, when Mary Breckinridge founded the Frontier Nursing Service in Kentucky (Frontier Nursing Service, n.d.). Over the ensuing decades, clinical nurse specialist and nurse practitioner roles developed. Today the concept of advanced practice nursing continues to evolve. As is true in other healthcare professions, prescribing is an important component of advanced nursing practice. However, achieving the right to prescribe has been challenging and is itself still in evolution.

Several factors underlie the uphill road to prescriptive authority for nursing: the primacy of physician practice, the public safety role of the states, policymakers' knowledge about advanced practice nursing, and nursing's ability to navigate political and legislative arenas. Each of these aspects, and their interplay, is key to understanding the current patchwork of prescriptive authority in the United States.

Prescription practice is relatively new. Prior to the twentieth century, pharmacists could dispense medications on consumer demand without consulting a physician. Over time, physicians gained dominance over prescriptive authority based on three factors: public safety regarding patent medicines, American Medical Association (AMA) ownership of "Ingredient Disclosure" and "Seal of Approval" designations, and pharmaceutical companies' realization that physicians could be used to market products (Harkless, 1989; Starr, 1982).

Physicians have had automatic prescriptive authority by virtue of their title and have not had to justify or prove competency to prescribe. Organized medicine via the AMA and state medical societies, however, persistently insists that other provider groups demonstrate their qualification (Sutliff, 1996). A variety of rules and limitations has been enacted in different states to regulate nurse prescription. Some states allow truly independent prescribing by the APN. Most require some sort of oversight, either through supervision or collaborative agreement. The AMA continues to insist that physicians retain responsibility for all patient care regardless of the setting, although evidence is lacking to justify this ultimate supervisory role for physicians (American Medical Association, n.d.).

Physicians have traditionally dominated public policymaking in health care, largely because theirs was the first recognized health profession and thus they were able to define healthcare practice. Beginning in 1721, physicians first sought licensure in the United States as a method of excluding competition from so-called empiricks and quacks. Formal licensure, undertaken by the medical society, was granted by Massachusetts in 1781, and by other states soon thereafter (Rothstein, 1985). However, it was not until the mid-1800s that a statutory definition of healing came into play, which placed diagnosis, treatment, surgery, and prescribing firmly in medicine's arena; by 1901, every state had adopted this approach (Starr, 1982). Thus, other healthcare professions were required to justify their inclusion in the "healing arts" or like statute to avoid violating prohibitions against the practice of medicine by nonphysicians (Safriet, 1992). Physician predominance spills over even now to popular culture, which often depicts physicians as the only available prescribers: "Ask your doctor about our new drug."

The perceived need to protect the public has likewise played an important role in whether prescriptive authority was granted to nurses. State legislators and other policymakers often raise the safety issue when debating prescriptive authority and other scope-of-practice concerns, largely because they lack knowledge about advanced nursing practice and education. Nurse practitioners have been studied virtually from the inception of their profession to ensure that patients would not be harmed under their care, and such studies continue to abound (Beck, 1995; Mundinger et al., 2000; Office of Technology Assessment, 1986). Every such study confirms that advanced practice nurses are safe, effective, and well-liked providers.

A third component contributing to the state of prescriptive authority for advanced practice is nursing's increasing understanding and involvement in the political process and policymaking. Understanding the context in which laws and regulations are made is crucial to implementing change. This includes understanding of not only the formal process of rule and law making but also the impact of campaign contributions, lobbying efforts, and public opinion.

Crafting laws and regulations is at once both formal and informal. The formality resides in the technical process. A proposed bill is introduced, generally to a subcommittee of the legislature. Frequently, testimony is heard from supporters and opponents of the bill, and at the state level, such hearings are usually open to public view. Lawmakers in the subcommittee then vote on the proposed bill. If approved, the bill issues to the full legislature for a vote. If passed by whatever majority the state requires, the bill goes to the governor for signature. Once signed, it becomes law as of the effective date named in the bill. If not signed (vetoed), the legislature might revote and, with a substantial majority, override the veto, in which case the bill becomes law.

The informal part of this process involves the human element: the lobbying effort, the personal experiences of the legislators around the topic of the bill, the campaign contributions from supporters or opponents, and the public's opinion on the bill's content. Even if the bill is well reasoned and articulate, a legislator may choose to vote against it because she thinks her constituents will not be happy if she votes in favor of passage, or because her own experiences lead her to distrust the outcome if the bill passed, or because she feels she owes a "no" vote to a major campaign contributor who opposes the bill or to a fellow legislator whose support she desires for her own proposed legislation.

Rule-making is also generally open to public view, but less directly. When an agency, such as a board of nursing, proposes a rule, the proposal is published in some sort of state register and indicates a window of time for the public or interested parties to comment. Sometimes opportunity to present testimony in person is offered, but frequently comments are submitted in writing. The agency reads and weighs the comments, and then either issues the rule or a revised rule or decides to withdraw the proposed rule.

As with legislation, rule-making also has its human element that influences the outcome. In addition, rule-making is in many ways less directly visible, and this can make it hard for nurses and other lay persons to access the rule-making process.

After nearly 4 decades of debate, prescriptive authority for advanced practice nurses exists almost universally in the United States. As of 2013, all states except Georgia recognize direct pre-scriptive authority for nurse practitioners (von Gizycki, 2013). In 2004, Georgia allowed APNs to phone in a prescription as a delegated medical act, but APNs are not still allowed to write prescriptions (Georgia Code Annotated, 2004). New Mexico, on the other hand, allows APNs fully independent practice, includ-ing full prescriptive rights (Nursing Practice Act, 1978). Only six states limit nurse prescription to legend (noncontrolled) drugs: Alabama, Florida, Georgia, Kentucky, Missouri, and Hawaii (Drug Enforcement Administration, 2005). All other states allow at least Schedule III–V prescribing by nurses (Towers, 2005).

DISCUSSION QUESTIONS

1. What does the restriction to Schedules III to V imply for practice? Consider that Ritalin (methylphenidate), fentanyl, and Demerol (meperidine) are categorized as Schedule II controlled substances.
2. What other concerns besides public safety might be at play in restricting nurse practitioner prescriptive authority?

Supervision, Collaboration, and Independent Practice

As mentioned earlier, many APNs practice under supervision or a collaborative agreement. How does supervision differ from col-laboration? In general terms, supervision seems to indicate more direct control of the nurse's practice by a physician, whereas a col-laborative arrangement indicates less oversight by the physician. Legally, however, the definitions of these terms are specific to each state, and there is no consistent usage among states.

Collaboration, especially, has many definitions and can look very similar to supervision. In Illinois, for example, APNs practice "in collaboration" with physicians under a written agreement that "shall authorize the categories of care, treatment, or procedures to be performed by the advanced practice nurse" (Nursing and Advanced Practice Act, 1999, Sec. 15-15). In Ohio, *collaboration* is defined as a "standard care arrangement" between a physician and a nurse, under which the physician is "continuously available to communicate with the nurse" (Nurse Practice Act, 2002, Sec. B). Connecticut defines *collaboration* as "a mutually agreed upon relationship" between a physician and an APN that "shall address a reasonable and appropriate level of consultation and referral, coverage for the patient in the absence of the advanced practice registered nurse, a method to review patient outcomes and a method of disclosure of the relationship to the patient" (Nursing, General Statutes of Connecticut, 2004, Sec. (b)). Some states, such as New York and Texas, define collaboration as practice under mandated written protocols devised by the physician (New York State Nurse Practice Act, 2005; Texas Statutes, 2005).

Another twist to nurse prescriptive authority is whether the nurse is limited to prescribing from some type of formulary. This may be in addition to the nurse's authority to prescribe only certain schedules of drugs. The formulary may consist of a list of the drug categories (or in some cases the actual medication names) the nurse is allowed to prescribe. Or it may simply list the categories or medications that are disallowed. Either way, it adds another layer of regulation. For example, in the state of New Hampshire APNs have independent practice but may prescribe only according to an exclusionary formulary that is established and reviewed by the Joint Health Council, which consists of members of the Board of Medicine (three members), Board of Pharmacy (two members), and Board of Nursing (three members).

Other limitations on the nurse's ability to prescribe may exist. In Texas, for instance, prescriptive authority is granted only to particular practice sites, such as community health centers, certain private physician practices, and rural practice sites (Texas Statutes, 2005). A nurse practitioner in California "does not have an additional scope of practice beyond the usual RN scope and must rely on standardized procedures for authorization to perform overlapping medical functions" (Terry, 2002). Nurse practitioners in Illinois, like those in several other states, are granted prescriptive authority as a delegation of medical care by a physician. The Illinois statute, however, specifically notes that the physician "may, but is not required to, delegate limited prescriptive authority to an advanced practice nurse" (Nursing and Advanced Practice Act, 1999, Sec. 15-20(a)).

DISCUSSION QUESTIONS

1. Explore the difference between supervision and collaboration, including the terms' legal definitions.
2. Why might legislators restrict advanced practice to a particular site or setting? What are the advantages and disadvantages of this arrangement?

CASE STUDIES

Why do APNs continue to practice under these restrictive arrangements? Consider the following three cases.

CASE 1: CONNECTICUT

Advanced practice nursing has been present in Connecticut since the late 1940s, both in training programs and practice. Clinical nurse specialists and nurse practitioners are governed as APNs under the same section of the Nurse Practice Act (Nursing, General Statutes of Connecticut, 2004). Certified nurse–midwives are governed by another statute and achieved prescriptive authority before APNs did.

In the mid-1980s, APNs functioned under the following practice act:

Sec. 20-871. Definition of nursing and practical nursing. (a) The practice of nursing by a registered nurse is defined as the process of diagnosing human responses to actual or potential health problems, providing supportive and restorative care, health counseling and teaching, case finding and referral, collaborating in the implementation of the total health care regimen and executing the medical regimen under the direction of a licensed physician or dentist.

A health maintenance organization (HMO) from another state wished to start business in Connecticut. This HMO relied on nurse practitioners with adequate prescriptive authority; otherwise, the HMO physicians would have to prescribe for their own and the nurse practitioners' patients, an inefficient and costly practice.

Early inquiries by the HMO established that nurse practitioners at a major hospital in Connecticut did prescribe directly. When the HMO raised APN prescriptive authority with the Department of Consumer Protection (DPC), however, it discovered that this prescribing arrangement was under informal and unwritten approval that had been granted by the DPC years earlier as part of its regulation of pharmacies. DPC now realized that APNs were practicing in many settings and that prescriptive authority was unclear.

When the state legislature addressed the issue the next year at the request of the DPC, it referred the issue to the state Department of Health (DOH), the licensure authority governing APNs and other clinicians, as a matter of regulating who can prescribe rather than prescribing per se. DOH formed a task force consisting of several physicians and APNs. Many meetings were held to explore the variety of advanced practice settings and activities; whether prescribing was an innate professional act or a delegated medical one; the virtues and deficits of formularies; the wisdom of limited prescriptive authority; whether APNs could or should dispense; what other models were used around the United States; whether different settings necessitated site-specific "guidance and control"; and whether APNs could have blanket authority to prescribe. In short, the coalition considered every convolution of the intersections of pharmacy, medicine, and nursing. Legislation eventually emerged in 1990 and a new license for advanced practice nursing was created. Advance practice nursing was addressed as

> [T]he performance of advanced level nursing practice activities which, by virtue of post-basic specialized education and experience, are appropriate to and may be performed by an advanced practice registered nurse. The advanced practice registered nurse performs acts of diagnosis and treatment of alterations in health status... [and may] under the direction of a physician licensed to practice in this state and in accordance

with written protocols, and if practicing in… a hospital, home for the aged, health care facility for the handicapped, nursing home, rest home, mental health facility, substance abuse treatment facility, infirmary operated by an educational institution for the care of students enrolled in, and faculty and staff of, such institution, or facility operated and maintained by any state agency and providing services for the prevention, diagnosis and treatment or care of human health conditions, or an industrial health facility… which serves at least two thousand employees, or a clinic operated by a state agency, municipality, or private nonprofit corporation, or a clinic operated by any educational institution prescribed by regulations adopted pursuant to said section, prescribe, dispense, and administer medical therapeutics and corrective measures, except that an APRN licensed pursuant to Section 3 of this Act and maintaining current certification from the American Association of Nurse Anesthetists who is prescribing and administering medical therapeutics during surgery may only do so if the physician who is medically directing the prescriptive activity is physically present in the institution, clinic, or other prescribed setting where such surgery is being performed.

APN prescriptive authority, though obtained from a separate license, was dependent on an approved site, under physician direction, with site-specific protocols listing the "medical therapeutics, corrective measures, laboratory tests, or other diagnostic procedures" that might be "prescribed, dispense or administered" by an APN in "various circumstances." Only Schedule IV and V medications (nonsteroidal anti-inflammatory drugs, mild steroid creams, and the like) could be prescribed.

As often happens, the reality of prescribing overwhelmed the legal framework under which APNs could prescribe. APNs continued to work in a variety of settings, increasing their scope of practice and prescribing appropriate to patient care. By the 1990s, virtually no physicians or APNs were following the mandated restrictions. And then, in 1997, another outside force caused the prescriptive authority to be reexamined.

Congress passed the 1997 Balanced Budget Act (BBA), including, for the first time ever, direct reimbursement to APNs under Medicare. The statute required, however, that a collaborative relationship exist between the APN and at least one physician. This raised concerns in states where

APNs practiced independently (10 at that time) and where APNs were still under direction or supervision—Connecticut being one.

The leadership of the state's APN group, to the surprise and consternation of other nursing leaders, arranged a loose coalition with the nurse psychotherapists, nurse anesthetists, and clinical nurse specialists to open the practice act for independent practice. The coalition at best was ill defined and ticklish, as was the strategy. Communication between the coalition parties was scant, and the Medical Society was never considered as a potential member. The entire episode ended with bitter and very acrimonious testimony from the Medical Society and the APN coalition's rejoinder, to the embarrassment of legislative sponsors. Just prior to a legislative decision to send the issue back to committee for more study, the bill was withdrawn. This effectively kept the issue under control of the APNs and the sponsors, providing anyone *would* sponsor a bill in a future session. (Otherwise, the issue would be sent immediately to committee, session after session, until someone felt like taking it to the floor.)

Despite the instincts of most nursing leaders to keep their heads down for future sessions, the BBA language virtually demanded another try. Therefore, the coalition gathered again, hardly more cohesive than before, but this time with a major strength. A well-known senator, herself a registered nurse (RN) and a savvy legislator with power over healthcare issues, agreed to make it a priority. The legislative arena was rife with healthcare issues regarding patient rights and the rights of physicians to organize, issues falling to the senator's committee. All told, the Medical Society watched 27 bills closely; only one of them concerned APNs, but all of them were in the senator's committee. The senator made it a condition of sponsorship that the coalition hammer out the details of the new prescriptive authority with the Medical Society before she would introduce it.

The coalition drafted a bill for consideration, reflecting independent practice based on national certification procedures (already required for APN licensure in Connecticut). Heavy emphasis was placed on the 1997 BBA language, which clearly recognized APN practice as legitimate and not needful of supervision. However, the federal language did invoke collaboration, not independence, and the Medical Society made much of this. Medicine did not push for an elaborate definition, however, and the APNs came to agree that collaboration would be acceptable for now.

The Medical Society wanted collaborative agreements to be in writing, but only for prescriptive authority, and still at the total discretion of all parties regarding the authority. No objection was raised to allowing APNs to prescribe Schedule II and Schedule III medications. The APNs agreed to the requirement for written collaboration for prescriptive practice.

The legislation issued to committee and to the full legislature with very little disturbance and with glowing statements of consensus from the Society and the various nursing groups. Regulations for APNs were eliminated (having merely echoed the now defunct law), which meant protocols were no longer needed. The direction clause in the nurse practice act was replaced with this language:

> The advanced practice nurse may, in collaboration with a physician licensed to practice in this state, prescribe, dispense, and administer medical therapeutics and corrective measures.... For purposes of this subsection, "collaboration" means a mutually agreed upon relationship between an advanced practice registered nurse and a physician who is educated, trained or has relevant experience that is related to the work of such APRN. The collaboration shall address a reasonable and appropriate level of consultation and referral, coverage for the patient in the absence of the APRN, a method to review patient outcomes, and a method of disclosure of the relationship to the patient. Relative to the exercise of prescriptive authority, the collaboration between an APRN and a physician shall be in writing and shall address the level of schedule II and III controlled substances that the ARPN may prescribe, including but not limited to, the review of medical therapeutics, corrective measures, laboratory tests and other diagnostic procedures that the APRN may prescribe, dispense and administer.

DISCUSSION QUESTIONS:

1. Discuss the difference between state statute and regulation.
2. What is the difference between prescribing as a "delegated medical act" and prescribing as an "innate quality of professional practice"?
3. Identify what "homework" APRNs should do prior to open discussions to change the state practice act.

4. Review how a bill becomes law and compare it to the process that occurred in Connecticut.

*****

CASE 2: MISSOURI

Missouri was the site of a case infamous in the early history of the nurse practitioner movement: *Sermchief v. Gonzales* (1983). This landmark case upheld the very existence of nurse practitioners, who had been sued by the state Medical Society for the illegal practice of medicine. The court upheld the legality of advanced practice, including prescriptive authority, noting the practice act required adequate education for nurses in such roles.

In 1987, Missouri passed a law under which physicians would be punished for "providing medication to a patient without first establishing a patient-physician relationship" (Sullivan, 1998, p. 328). The law was intended to prevent prescriptions for oneself, friends, or family. The Missouri Board of Healing Arts, however, interpreted the new law to mean that nurse practitioners could not prescribe medication for any patients without a physician first examining the patient.

The board investigated pharmacies and physicians who allowed nurse practitioners to prescribe without the requisite a priori physician examination for possible disciplinary action. Not surprisingly, physicians and pharmacies immediately stopped working with nurse practitioners. With this interpretation, the board unilaterally amended the nurse practice act.

Despite many attempts by a multidisciplinary coalition to remedy this situation, the practice environment was not changed until 1993, when the Missouri legislature passed a law establishing collaborative nurse–physician relationships. It left interpretation of the definition of collaboration with the Board of Healing Arts, and subsequent administrative interpretation was contentious. The law stated that the physician delegated medical authority in the collaborative agreement, including the right to prescribe. However, nurse practitioners were able to prescribe without first having the patient seen by a physician (Sullivan, 1998).

In 1996, 3 years after the collaborative law, regulations governing collaboration were issued. The collaborative agreement was required to be written and contain "disease specific protocols with clear criteria for making the diagnosis" (Rathbun & Richards, 1997). APNs were not allowed to prescribe controlled substances.

An article written by a physician and a lawyer to educate physicians and nurses about the new regulations advised that the agreement contain a formulary with specific drugs listed. "Deciding what is the 'appropriate hypertensive' is a pharmacology course, not a standing order" (Rathbun & Richards, 1997, p. 4). The article estimated that a family nurse practitioner would need "50 to 100 protocols to work from" (Rathbun & Richards, 1997, p. 4). It is not known how influential this advice was.

In 2004, the APNs in Missouri proposed a bill to grant them the right to prescribe controlled substances if permitted under a collaborative agreement (Crouse, 2005). The bill failed, and the issue was raised again in 2005. It did not pass.

DISCUSSION QUESTIONS:

1. How did prescriptive authority originally undergo revision in Missouri?

2. Identify future APN issues similar to that of prescriptive authority that may arise and how you would begin to address those issues.

3. Discuss the arguments for and against APN prescriptive authority for controlled substances.

*****

CASE 3: GEORGIA

Georgia is the only state that does not allow APNs to write prescriptions. APNs may, under physician approval, phone in a prescription. However, not all pharmacies allow nonwritten prescriptions; the VA, for instance, requires written prescriptions. Some private medical facilities recognize that telephonic prescriptions lead to errors and require written prescriptions to be issued.

This is the case at the large group practice at Memorial Health University Medical in Savannah, Georgia. APNs there work under a policy that patients must leave with a written prescription in hand. This means APNs must track down a doctor with time to write a prescription before patients can leave the clinic. "This definitely increases patient wait time and ultimately decreases the number of patients I can see due to lost time," said an APN working there (Hart, personal communication, February 28, 2005). Neither patients nor APNs are happy with the situation (Hart, personal communication, February 28, 2005). In other settings, patients often have to wait while an APN finds time between patients to make the call. Otherwise, the patient has to wait until the physician can write out and sign the prescription. This can cause a great delay, sometimes days from the actual visit (Hart, personal communication, February 23, 2008).

It is not for lack of trying that the APNs find themselves excluded from a basic piece of practice. Over the last 11 years, they have proposed legislation each year to change the law, and each time the powerful Medical Association of Georgia (MAG) manages to keep the bill in committee or to actually defeat it if issued to the general legislature. Even MAG recognizes the absurdity of allowing APNs to "recommend" a medication but not to actually prescribe it. The executive director of MAG has said the practice is "illogical." However, MAG continues to adhere to the belief that physicians must be involved in any prescribing (Jones, personal communication, February 28, 2005).

The issue of nurse prescribing has a long history in Georgia, and several twists may explain the current dilemma. In 1979, the state's attorney general issued an opinion that it was legal under the nurse practice act for nurses to "prescribe" under written protocols from a physician. The practice, developed nearly 20 years earlier, was essential to 245 rural public health clinics and numerous public health, homeless, and other clinics across the state that had trouble hiring sufficient numbers of physicians (A. Hill, personal communication, February 4, 1989). In fact, most physicians were usually contracted not to be on site, but to be available for nurse consultation as needed (McCarthy, personal communication, June 15, 1988). The attorney general's opinion clarified that public health nurses were legally capable of prescribing birth control pills and antibiotics under written protocols for the impoverished patients whose only medical care occurs in a public health clinic.

In 1988, for reasons unknown now, the issue rose again. The director of the Drugs and Narcotics Agency in Georgia, which regulates prescribing practices, asked the attorney general to reexamine the practice of nurse prescription under protocol. This time, the attorney general found that the practice was illegal. "Nurses may not write or telephone in prescriptions by referring to a written protocol" (McCarthy, personal communication, August 2, 1988). The rural public health clinics were, however, still dependent on this model because too few physicians were willing to practice in those areas. The fallout from the sudden finding that nurses could not, in fact, prescribe under protocol was immediate and urgent.

The directors of the 19 public health districts sought and gained a meeting with the commissioner of Public Health to assess what options might be available so patient care would not be compromised. There did not seem to be many: either the physicians' fees for overseeing prescribing were too steep, or there simply were no physicians in a particular health district who could be contracted to "prescribe." The commissioner wrote to the attorney general asking for further clarification of the opinion, pointing out the circumstances and history of the protocol system, and summarizing the literature on the safety of such arrangements. Meanwhile, the public health nurses were forced to call the backup physicians "for every single thing" covered by protocol to comply with the new opinion. One nurse observed, "It makes more work and it's time consuming, but we're doing it so we won't be in violation of the law. We're really trying to avoid sending people to the emergency room for their medications" (McCarthy, personal communication, August 2, 1988).

Two months later, the attorney general wrote back to the commissioner of Public Health and affirmed that his opinion forbade nurses from prescribing in any manner. "Under Georgia law, the medication decision must be made by a physician," he found, and "that is as clear as a bell" (McCarthy, personal communication, October 5, 1988). The commissioner responded that his office would seek legislative remedy in the next session, and in the meantime he would work to alleviate the burden on the poor who frequent the public health clinics (McCarthy, personal communication, October 5, 1988).

The commissioner was successful in his legislative approach, and the governor signed a new law that explicitly allowed nurses to prescribe. The commissioner was joined in his efforts by the Georgia Nurses' Association and a state senator who recognized the gist of the problem as "a turf struggle" (Hill, personal communication, February 4, 1989). Although the physician and pharmacy lobbies raised strong objections, the legislature recognized the tremendous burden on patients and the fact that the "system came to a very, very slow crawl," as observed by the nurses' attorney (Hill, personal communication, February 4, 1989).

In 1994, the nurses proposed legislation to allow nurses with advanced training to prescribe medications directly. This effort, as well as the one in the following year, failed to create a bill. In 1996, however, the nurses got both a bill and a lot of good publicity. The failure of the 1996 effort did not deter the APNs from trying again the next year. As before, the papers followed the debate and endorsed the nurses. MAG raised the usual arguments of insufficient training and physician supremacy. MAG also noted its fear that the health maintenance organizations (HMOs) designed to cut costs would hire nurse practitioners over physicians if nurse practitioners could prescribe. The 1997 effort failed to produce legislation.

By 2005, MAG admitted that the main concern was the issue of collaboration, which to MAG "implies nurses are equal to physicians," causing safety problems for patients (Hart, personal communication, February 23, 2005). The nurses have stated that they are willing to accept prescribing under supervision (Hart, personal communication, February 23, 2005). Nonetheless, in 2005 the MAG website (http://www.mag.org) urges physicians to call legislators and ask for a negative vote because of public safety issues. Once again, APNs were denied prescriptive authority.

DISCUSSION QUESTIONS:

1. Discuss the merits of the various arguments used against APN prescriptive authority in Georgia.

2. The Georgia APN community has excelled at public news coverage for their cause. What other options exist?

3. Discuss whether advanced practice nurses are undertrained, or whether physicians in certain settings are overtrained.

References

American Medical Association. (n.d.). Guidelines for integrated practice of physician and nurse practitioner. Retrieved from http://www.ama-assn.org/resources/doc/PolicyFinder/policyfiles/HnE/H-160.950.HTM

Beck, M. (1995). Improving America's health care: Authorizing independent prescriptive privileges for advanced practice nurses. University of San Francisco Law Review, 29(95), 1–998.

Crouse, A. (2005). Missouri state senate. Retrieved from http://www.senate.mo.gov/05info/BTS_Web/Bill.aspx?SessionType=R&BillID=65

Drug Enforcement Administration. (2005). Mid-level practitioners (MLP) authorization by state. Retrieved from http://www.deadiversion.usdoj.gov/drugreg/practioners/

Frontier Nursing Service. (n.d.). How FNS began: A brief history of the Frontier Nursing Service. Retrieved from http://www.frontiernursing.org/History/HowFNSbegan.shtm

Georgia Code Annotated, Title 43, Section 34-26.1(8). (2004). Retrieved from http://law.justia.com/codes/georgia/2010/title-43/chapter-34/article-2/43-34-26-1

Harkless, G. (1989). Prescriptive authority: Debunking common assumptions. *Nurse Practitioner, 14*, 57–61.

Mundinger, M. O., Kane, R. L., Lenz, E., Totten, A. M., Tsai, W.-Y, Cleary, P. D.,... Shelanski, M. L. (2000). Primary care outcomes in patients treated by nurse practitioners or physicians. *Journal of the American Medical Association, 283*(1), 59–68.

New York State Nurse Practice Act, New York State Consolidated Laws, Chapter 16, Article 139, Section 6900 *et seq.* (2005). Retrieved from http://www.op.nysed.gov/prof/nurse/article139.htm

Nurse Practice Act, Ohio Revised Code 4723-9-01, *et seq.* (2002). Retrieved from http://codes.ohio.gov/oac/4723-9

Nursing, General Statutes of Connecticut, Ch 378, Sec. 20-87(a) (2004). Retrieved from http://www.cga.ct.gov/2011/pub/chap378.htm

Nursing and Advanced Practice Act. 225 Illinois Compiled Statutes 65/15-1, *et seq.* (1999). Retrieved from http://www.ilga.gov/legislation/ilcs/ilcs3.asp?ActID=1312&ChapterID=24

Nursing Practice Act. (1995). Missouri Revised Statutes, 334.104.1. Retrieved from http://www.moga.mo.gov/statutes/chapters/chap335.htm

Nursing Practice Act. (1978). New Mexico Statutes Annotated, Chapter 61, Article 3-1 *et seq.* Retrieved from http://public.nmcompcomm.us/nmpublic/gateway.dll/?f=templates&fn=default.htm

Office of Technology Assessment, U.S. Congress. (1986). *Nurse practitioners, physician assistants, and certified nurse-midwives: A policy analysis (Health Technology Case Study*

37), OTA-HCS-37. Washington, DC: U.S. Government Printing Office.

Rathbun, K. C., & Richards, E. P. (1997). Supervising RNs and advance practice nurses: New regulations for Missouri. *Missouri Medicine, 94,* 17. Retrieved from http://biotech.law.lsu.edu/Articles/apn.html

Rothstein, W. (1985). *American physicians in the 19th century: From sects to science.* Baltimore, MD: Johns Hopkins University Press.

Safriet, B. (1992). Health care dollars and regulatory sense: The role of advanced practice nursing. *Yale Journal of Regulation, 9,* 417–487.

Sermchief v. Gonzales, 660 S.W.2d 683 (Mo. 1983).

Starr, P. (1982). *The social transformation of American medicine.* New York, NY: Basic Books.

Sullivan, T. (1998). *Collaboration: A health care imperative.* New York, NY: McGraw-Hill.

Sutliff, L. (1996). Myth, mystique and monopoly in the prescription of medicine. *Nurse Practitioner, 21*(3), 153–155.

Terry, R. (2002). The certified nurse practitioner. Retrieved from http://www.rn.ca.gov/pdfs/regulations/npr-b-23.pdf

Texas Statutes. (2005). Occupations Code. Title 3. Health Professions. Subtitle E. Regulation of Nursing. Chapter 301. Nurses. Retrieved from http://codes.lp.findlaw.com/txstatutes/OC/3/E

Towers, J. (2005). After forty years. *Journal of the American Academy of Nurse Practitioners, 17*(1), 9.

von Gizycki, D. (2013). APRN prescribing law: A state-by-state summary. Retrieved from http://www.medscape.com/viewarticle/440315

Additional Resources

Gregory, L. (2004, February 3). Nurses may get green light to write prescriptions. *Cedartown* (Georgia) *Standard,* p. 1.

Hadley, H. (1989). Nurses and prescriptive authority: A legal and economic analysis. *American Journal of Law and Medicine, 15*, 245–299.

Hanson, C. (2000). Understanding the regulatory and credentialing requirements for advanced practice nursing. In A. B. Hamric, J. A. Spross, & C. M. Hanson (Eds.), *Advanced nursing practice* (2nd ed., pp. 557–578). Philadelphia, PA: Saunders.

O'Brien, J. (2003). How nurse practitioners obtained provider status: Lessons for pharmacists. *American Journal Health-System Pharmacists, 62*(22), 2301–2307.

CHAPTER 4

Credentialing and Privileging

Lynette Hamlin, PhD, RN, CNM, FACNM

Learning Objectives

At the completion of this chapter, you will be able to:

1. Differentiate between credentialing and privileging.
2. Identify key players in your practice environment.
3. List the steps to obtain clinical privileges in a healthcare institution.
4. Identify the necessary paperwork in preparing your portfolio.
5. Discuss the obstacles and opportunities involved with establishing a practice base.

This case illustrates the trials and tribulations of beginning a practice, obtaining hospital privileges, and becoming credentialed with managed care organizations. It is also about identifying a community need for a service, identifying key players within organizations, and just plain schmoozing.

Part I: Background

This case occurs in a state where at the time advanced practice nurses and nurse–midwives practiced under their nursing license. There were no advanced practice laws, but the proposals for a law were on the table. The setting is the land of major pharmaceutical companies and a large military base. Five hospitals serve this area, each distinctly different, but all competing for beds and business. Surgi-centers and satellite facilities that contain health clubs, labs, and physician offices were moving into each other's "territory." The sociodemographics and economics of the community range from the uninsured melting pot to an area referred to as the Gold Coast.

Two hospitals are directly in the area of the Gold Coast, one hospital is on its fringes in the most rapidly growing area of the community, and two hospitals serve primarily the uninsured and the underinsured. In this county, the population segment with the largest growth in uninsured and underinsured individuals is Mexican immigrants, many of whom are unregistered aliens who migrated to the area for farm work. The Gold Coast hospitals advertise primary care and board-certified physicians. The two hospitals serving the poor and working poor have primarily non-board-certified physicians. In the area of obstetrics, most of the non-board-certified physicians work in solo practices, and the majority of board-certified obstetricians/gynecologists work in group practices.

The central repository for health care for the uninsured is the County Health Department. It operates a main clinic and several satellite clinics, providing primary care, family planning, and prenatal services. One physician, one certified nurse–midwife, and one nurse practitioner staff the family planning and prenatal clinics. The Health Department is funded by grants and county taxes. None of the physicians in the county provide prenatal care for uninsured women, and they also do not allow the Health Department providers to have hospital privileges to provide full-scope care. Instead, the women are seen prenatally at the Health Department, and when they begin labor they are walk-ins at the local hospitals, cared for by the hospital's on-call Ob/Gyn; the delivering physician bills for the maternity cycle care. Recently, Dr. Mays, a physician from the community who mostly serves the poor, began staffing some of the Health Department prenatal clinics. He then can admit maternity patients to his private practice when the women begin labor. This physician is the only physician in the area in a group practice in which all the partners are board certified.

Part II: Lisa

Lisa is an RN who works labor and delivery and postpartum at one of the Gold Coast hospitals. This hospital has the busiest labor and delivery unit in the county, and it is growing by leaps and bounds. Lisa is also a student in a nurse–midwifery program. For her clinical rotation in family planning she is assigned to be with the certified nurse–midwife (CNM) at the Health Department's family planning clinic. There are two other CNMs in the county, but they work as nurse educators in physician practices. No CNM has ever had privileges at any of the five hospitals in the county.

As Lisa is finishing her midwifery program, she decides that she would like to practice in this community—the community where she has lived her entire life. She enjoys the atmosphere of the hospital where she works and decides to pursue a practice in that setting. This project is three-pronged: determining the need for a nurse–midwifery practice, finding a supervising physician (this state does not have independent APN practice), and finding a hospital to obtain privileges.

Lisa begins to assess the community's need and openness to a nurse–midwifery practice. First, she becomes active in the American College of Nurse–Midwives, the professional organization for CNMs. She joins the national committee that works on practice issues and restriction of practice issues. Lisa finds this an excellent opportunity to learn, network, and develop support systems to help her reach her goal.

Lisa then contacts women's organizations in the community. She presents at mothers' clubs, library groups, and La Leche League meetings. She finds women very receptive to the idea of nurse-midwifery care. Some women who moved to this community from other areas where they were cared for by nurse–midwives state that they would really like that option here.

Lisa begins to write letters to the hospitals in the community asking for an application for privileges. Each hospital administrator writes back to say that the hospital does not have a category for midwives, it does not see a need for these services, and its strategic plan focuses on the growth of primary care services (see **Figures 4-1** and **4-2**). In a conversation with the vice president at her current employer, the vice president states that the hospital is known for having an all-board-certified staff and it has no intention of changing that.

Simultaneously, Lisa begins to meet with area physicians. Some are receptive to nurse-midwifery and would like to see that service provided at their hospital, but they state they are unwilling to "take up that fight" with their hospital at this time. Meanwhile, Lisa works with her professional association's attorney, who writes to her employer (see **Figure 4-3**).

DISCUSSION QUESTIONS

1. Think about the communities where you have lived. Was there access to advanced practice nurses? Why or why not?

2. What resources are available in your professional organization to help you in establishing a practice?

3. What other community or hospital resources could you utilize in your quest to establish a practice?

4. Which hospital committees and key players have a role in determining medical staff privileges?

5. What does the Joint Commission *Medical Staff Handbook* say about privileges for advanced practice nurses and CNMs?

6. What documentation should Lisa be keeping through this process?

June 24, Year 1

Ms. Lisa, RN
111 Lake Road
Gold Coast, IL

Dear Ms. Lisa:

I am writing in response to your June 19 letter regarding your continued interest in obtaining nonmedical professional staff privileges here at Gold Coast Hospital. Although I recognize your interest in providing independent nurse-midwifery services here at the hospital, a clear need for these services has not been established by the Board at this time. The Medical Staff Development Committee of the Board, which oversees the responsibility of determining need for medical practitioners at Gold Coast Hospital, recently discussed the overall issue of the utilization of physician extenders at the hospital. The committee has recommended that the primary need and focus for medical staff development at this time is in the primary care specialties of internal medicine and family practice. As in the past, the Staff Development Committee will periodically review the need for medical and nonmedical professional staff.

Thank you for your continued interest in Gold Coast Hospital. Please feel free to contact us in the future should you maintain an interest in the hospital.

Sincerely yours,
Jane Smith

Executive Vice President, Gold Coast Hospital

FIGURE 4-1   Letter from hospital.

February 14, Year 2

Ms. Lisa, RN
111 Lake Road
Gold Coast, IL

Dear Ms. Lisa:

The purpose of this correspondence is to respond to your letter of December 14 to Dr. Min, President of the Medical Staff. In this letter, you requested admitting and obstetrical privileges at Vulnerable Hospital within the scope of your license as a certified nurse–midwife. (As you are probably aware, we are not required under state or federal law to extend privileges to any or all independent practitioners, irrespective of whether they qualify as Medical Staff Members or as allied health practitioners.) At this time, we do not extend such privileges to nurse–midwives nor do we perceive a need for these services in our community.

We will keep your letter and the information you provided on file should the Board of Directors at some later point in time decide to raise the question of whether to grant clinical privileges to nurse–midwives.

Again, thank you for your interest in Vulnerable Hospital.

Sincerely,
Amy Smith

President, Vulnerable Hospital

FIGURE 4-2   Letter from hospital.

August 2, Year 2

Mr. President
Gold Coast Hospital

Re: Clinical Privileges for Nurse–Midwives

Dear Mr. President:

I am the general counsel of the American College of Nurse–Midwives ("ACNM"), the national professional organization of certified nurse–midwives ("CNMs") in the United States. I am writing to you because it is the policy of ACNM and its Board of Directors that CNMs should be able to practice and provide nurse-midwifery services in all practice settings and should be able to obtain clinical privileges to provide nurse-midwifery services in hospitals. I have been informed by one of our members that Gold Coast Hospital has not only been unreceptive to her request to obtain an application for clinical privileges at your institution but has delayed in even providing the application form.

If the information I have been provided with is accurate, the exclusion of CNMs as a class from Gold Coast Hospital is very troubling. A decision by a group of competitors, such as a clinical department of a hospital or the executive committee of a medical staff acting on behalf of that staff, to exclude an entire category of competing non-MD health professionals has been determined, in various federal court and agency decisions, to be a violation of the federal antitrust laws.

The Federal Trade Commission, which has a strong record of enforcement of the antitrust laws and policies of the United States in the health care market, has filed a number of complaints against hospital medical staffs which have taken actions such as barring an entire category of health professionals, such as CNMs, or dragging their feet in credentialing a group of physicians who practice in a particular competitive manner, such as HMO employees. Private actions filed by nonphysician health professionals have been successful, as the enclosed decision in *Oltz V. St. Peter's Community Hospital* also demonstrates.

FIGURE 4-3 Attorney's letter to employer.   (*Continued*)

I would be glad to work with your counsel on these matters and to help educate administrative staff on the process of credentialing CNMs, since these are issues on which my colleagues and I at ACNM have particular experience. Please see the enclosed article on vicarious liability, which was published in the March–April 1994 *Journal of Nurse-Midwifery*; I can also provide, if you so request, a copy of a Journal article on the mechanics and underlying clinical issues involved in credentialing nurse–midwives.

I must also inform you that it is the policy of ACNM and its Board to notify appropriate governmental enforcement authorities regarding barriers to practice encountered by our members. Attorneys at the Federal Trade Commission and Department of Justice have publicly indicated their interest in learning about class-based exclusion of cost-effective non-MD providers such as CNMs as the result of concerted action by groups of physicians. State attorneys general have also indicated their interest in making the health care services market in their respective states a strong and competitive one.

I would hope that this problem could be resolved promptly in the best interests of Gold Coast Hospital, CNMs in the Gold Coast area, and consumers of health care services in your community. If I can be of any assistance, or if you wish to obtain any additional information, please do not hesitate to contact me or have your attorneys do so. The ACNM staff is dedicated to assisting hospitals, managed care plans, and other institutional entities in the health care market to learn more about the effective inclusion of nurse-midwifery services. I look forward to hearing from your institution.

Very truly yours,

General Counsel

Cc: Dr. H, MD, Chair, Ob/Gyn Department

Staff Attorney, Federal Trade Commission

Office of State Attorney General

FIGURE 4-3 Attorney's letter to employer.

Part III: Success

When Lisa graduates from the nurse-midwifery program she continues to work at the same hospital as a staff RN and also works per diem at the Health Department family planning and prenatal clinics as a CNM. The staff at the Health Department encourage her to talk to the new physician in the community (Dr. Mays, the one in group practice), who staffs the clinics part time. They believe he would be receptive to a nurse–midwife. So, Lisa writes him a letter (**Figure 4-4**) and calls his office to make an appointment to meet with him. Dr. Mays's group practice includes three other physicians and two women's health nurse practitioners (who do not have hospital privileges).

Dr. Mays returns Lisa's phone call. During their meeting, he tells her that he worked with CNMs during his residency and they taught him most of what he knows. He also says that he went to medical school in Mexico and that his wife is a Mexican citizen. He says he feels a strong need to serve the immigrant Mexican population in this community. His dream is to grow a midwifery service within his practice that would eventually serve all of the women currently being seen in the disjointed system of the Health Department. Because many of his clients are Mexican, he attempts to hire only bilingual healthcare providers, and the majority of his staff are members of the Mexican community.

Dr. Mays and Lisa develop a practice agreement. The next step is to obtain hospital privileges. Dr. Mays practices at two hospitals. Because any hospital that grants a nurse–midwife staff privileges will initially require a physician to be present during the birth, he decides to put privileges forward at St. Bernadette's Hospital, where he has an office on campus. Also, in its bylaws St. Bernadette's Hospital has a medical staff category for allied health staff, so Dr. Mays knows the hospital cannot deny the application.

As word of this travels among the medical community, the Ob/Gyns in solo practice at St. Bernadette's Hospital are not happy. They call a meeting of the Department of Ob/Gyn Executive Committee, and Dr. Mays invites Lisa to attend this meeting.

June 1, Year 1

Dr. Mays
111 County Road
Gold Coast, IL

Dear Dr. Mays:

I am a certified nurse–midwife who is establishing a private practice in the County area. I believe there is a need and a desire for nurse-midwifery care in our community and I am excited to be at the forefront of its introduction. The American College of Nurse-Midwives and American College of Obstetricians and Gynecologists have developed a practice statement establishing avenues for referral and consultation. I need to establish a contractual relationship with a physician to ensure continuity of care for at-risk clients. I am currently in the process of requesting hospital privileges for obstetrical services at St. Bernadette's Hospital.

To introduce myself and some of my credentials to you, I am enclosing my resume for your review. Also, I would be more than willing to meet with the Department of Obstetrics and Gynecology Medical Staff at St. Bernadette's Hospital and perhaps others who would be in contact with CNM care to discuss the goals and philosophy of nurse-midwifery care. I would like to schedule a meeting with you to further discuss the potential for a collaborative practice agreement and how a collaborative relationship will benefit both of our practices.

If you have any questions please do not hesitate to contact me. I will contact your office to schedule an appointment.

Sincerely,

Lisa, CNM, RN

Enclosures

FIGURE 4-4   Letter to physician.

Prior to the meeting, Dr. Mays and Lisa work with legal counsel to anticipate potential roadblocks. One of the prep talks involved antitrust legislation.

An administrator from St. Bernadette's also attends the department meeting. He tells the physicians that there is a category in the medical staff for allied health professionals, so the physicians cannot block the appointment, but as members of the department, they can determine how and what the CNM can practice. The physicians decide to require that Dr. Mays be in attendance for all of Lisa's births. One physician remarks to Dr. Mays that she does not know how he will be able to afford a CNM when he has to attend all of the CNM's births. Dr. Mays and Lisa look at one another, and Dr. Mays tells this physician that because she brought up money she can no longer vote on this topic (read: antitrust prep).

After the meeting, Lisa prepares her materials for credentialing and privileging. (See **Figure 4-5**.) She also works with Dr. Mays's office manager to complete applications for credentialing with the insurers.

DISCUSSION QUESTIONS

1. What are common types of medical staff membership categories that are used for advanced practice nurses?

2. What advanced practice documents are important to organize prior to the process of establishing a practice?

3. What documents are needed for hospital and managed care applications?

4. What is a UPIN and what is it used for?

5. What is delineation of privileges and how often are privileges typically renewed?

A. Resume

B. Credentialing Materials

1. Nursing program transcript

2. ACC Certificate

3. Midwifery license

4. Nursing license (where applicable)

5. DEA certificate

6. State controlled substance license

7. Copy of CEU certificates

C. Academic Summary

1. Final statistics

2. Summary of clinical sites

   a. Name of site and dates of assignment

   b. Type of experience (antepartum, gynecological, primary care, intrapartum, full-scope)

   c. Brief summary of site: Sociodemographics of clients, type of midwifery service, service setting

3. Copy of graduate program Final Summary

FIGURE 4-5 Professional portfolio template.

BOX 4-1: *Credentialing and Privileges Tutorial*

Credentialing
- The process of assessing and validating the qualifications of a practitioner to provide member health services in a healthcare network and/or its components

Privileging
- The authorization granted to a practitioner by the healthcare network to provide specific patient care services. The services must fall within defined limits based on the practitioner's qualifications and current competence.

Documentation
- Documentation

   - Document every step of the process
   - Retain at least one copy of application, attachments, every letter, note, set of minutes, and other documents
   - Keep a journal or diary of the process for chronological accounting: meetings, phone calls
   - Request written notice and confirmation, not verbal
   - Follow up all conversations with a confirmatory letter

Key Players
- Hospital administration

   - Chief executive officer
   - CEO administrative assistant
   - Medical staff secretary
   - Medical staff chief
   - VP for nursing services
   - Board of trustees
   - Legal department
   - Medical records department

Medical Staff and Committees
- Chief of staff
- Bylaws committee

(Continued)

- Credentials committee
- Executive committee
- Clinical departments
- Quality assurance

Community Members
- Client base
- Potential clients
- Community residents
- Special interest groups
- Media

Establish Credibility
- Identify how key players perceive CNMs/APNs
- Identify sources of support and opposition; go beyond obstetrics community
- Use contacts: Clients, health educators, nurses, doulas, etc.
- Involve the professional community: Local chapter, individual CNMs/ APNs

Two Paths
- LIPs: Licensed independent practitioners can be credentialed through medical staff bylaws
- Non-LIPs: Can be credentialed through human resources policies or medical staff process

Medical Staff Membership
- Independent: Authorized to admit patients
- Dependent: May admit patients through physician; have delivery privileges
- Courtesy: May access patients' medical records

Membership Categories
- Medical staff
- Allied health
- Medical assistant
- Nursing
- Other

Process

- Obtain an application for privileges
- Organize practice documents

  - State laws and regulations
  - Including prescriptive authority
  - Practice guidelines
  - Any relevant clinical agreements with physician
  - Reimbursement policies of insurers

Documentation Continued

- Pertinent medical practice laws and regulations
- State hospital codes
- Laws/regulations relating to admitting or other privileges for APNs/CNMs or all non-MDs
- State laws with provisions for admission history and physical exam by CNMs/APNs
- Current edition of Joint Commission *Medical Staff Handbook*

Privileging Process

- Preapplication preparations

  - Obtain a copy of the medical staff bylaws
    - Where is the category for CNMs/APNs?
    - If not mentioned or non-MD category that precludes admitting privileges or medical staff membership—bylaws change

Finalize Plans with Collaborating Physician

- Identify
- Develop a plan of action
- Discuss key players and steps of the privileging process
- Identify any areas of concern for either party
- Brainstorm

Documents for the Application

- The Joint Commission requires confirmation from the original source!
- RN license
- APN/Midwifery license

(Continued)

- American College of Nurse–Midwives/ACNM Certification Council/ American Nurses Credentialing Center certification
- Academic transcripts
- Letters of reference

Documents

- Letter of support from collaborating physician
- Certificate of professional liability insurance
- Documentation of continuing education
- Recent physical exam
- Practice guidelines for inpatient care

Delineation of Privileges

- List of possible functions and procedures considered appropriate by the department
- Are you qualified?

Renewal of Privileges

- Typically every 2 years
- Continuing education
- Attendance at staff meetings

Duties of Ancillary Categories

- Decision of privileges may be made with department chair
- May not have complete due process protection
- May be nonvoting members of the department

Part IV: Establishing Credibility and Garnering Publicity

Lisa's application for privileges at St. Bernadette's Hospital and her managed care credentialing happened without a hitch. Then came Lisa's first day on call. Two of Dr. Mays's partners refused to take call with Lisa, so Dr. Mays volunteered to cover call so that Lisa could begin attending births as soon as possible. One morning at 5:00 a.m. Lisa received a call from Dr. Mays—there were two women in labor.

When Lisa and Dr. Mays arrived on labor and delivery, the nurses and physician partner going off-shift all said "good luck" but with sarcasm. One of the laboring women's screams was filling the labor floor. This hospital did not have access to round-the-clock anesthesia services, so an epidural was not available to her. She was a CHAMPUS patient and had had an epidural with her first child—this was her second. Lisa immediately went and sat with the woman and her screams stopped. The nurses on the unit called Lisa a miracle worker. Meanwhile, another woman in labor was admitted. It looked like Lisa's first day was going to be busy!

All three women birthed without complications and with Dr. Mays in attendance. Of course there were some kinks to work out between Lisa and the nursing staff—lights on, lights off, hands and knees position, supine position. Dr. Mays supported all of Lisa's decisions.

Afterward, Lisa and Dr. Mays worked with St. Bernadette's public relations department. Within a week the county newspaper ran a front-page story titled "Opening Doors: Recent Births May Mean More Midwives in the Delivery Room." A large photo of Lisa, the formerly screaming woman, and her baby also appeared on the front page of the newspaper. The woman was quoted as saying she would never have another child without a midwife.

In addition to supporting Lisa with hospital privileges, Dr. Mays began to move forward with his plan to care for more vulnerable women. By this time Lisa was faculty in a midwifery program and brought students with her to the office practice. Dr. Mays opened his hospital office once a week for Lisa and students to see clinic patients. Midwifery was well on its way in this county.

Bibliography

American College of Nurse–Midwives. (2012, May 12). Memo to members of the American College of Nurse–Midwives. Retrieved from http://www.midwife.org/ACNM/files/ccLibraryFiles/Filename/000000002126/Memo%20on%20Final%20CMS%20Rule%20on%20Medicare%20CoPs%20May%202012.pdf

American Nurses Association. (2010). APRNs with NPIs: Distribution by role and state. *ANA Issue Brief.* Retrieved from http://nursingworld.org/mainmenucategories/policy-advocacy/positions-and-Resolutions/Issue-Briefs/APRNs-with-NPIs.pdf

Harbison, S. (2003). APRNs and multi-state licensure compacts. *Journal of Pediatric Health Care, 17*(6), 321–323.

Joint Commission. (2011). *The medical staff handbook: A guide to Joint Commission standards* (3rd ed.). Oakbrook Terrace, IL: Author.

Kleinpell, R., Hravnak, M., Hinch, B., & Llewellyn, J. (2008). Developing an advanced practice nursing credentialing model for acute care facilities. *Nursing Administration Quarterly, 32*(4), 279–287.

Madgic, K., & Hravnak, M. (2005). Credentialing for nurse practitioners. *AACN Advanced Critical Care, 16*(1), 15–22.

Miller, S. (2000, May). Obtaining hospital privileges. *Patient Care for the Nurse Practitioner*, 84–87.

National Council of State Boards of Nursing. (2008). *Consensus model for APRN regulation: Licensure, accreditation, certification, and education.* Retrieved from http://www.aacn.nche.edu/education-resources/APRNReport.pdf

Summers, L. (2012, April–May–June). Clinical privileges: Opening doors for APRNs. *South Carolina Nurse*, 8.

CHAPTER 5

Managed Care, Healthcare Financial Management, and Reimbursement

Julie C. Jacobson Vann, PhD, MS, RN

Learning Objectives

At the completion of this chapter, you will be able to:

1. Compare and contrast the distinguishing operating characteristics of traditional health maintenance organizations, preferred provider organizations, exclusive provider organizations, and primary care case management programs with respect to gatekeeper mechanisms, coverage for in-network and out-of-network services, and utilization management mechanisms.
2. Critique the types of managed care delivery systems with respect to focus on quality of care and improving the health status of enrolled populations.
3. Describe the uninsured population in the United States, and analyze the implications for the healthcare delivery system.

4. Propose a healthcare systems strategy for addressing access-to-care issues for uninsured women needing services related to breast and/or cervical cancer.

5. Identify the funding challenges faced by advanced practice nurses and community-based providers in developing and sustaining health programs.

6. Evaluate the alternative strategies that may be currently available to fund nursing-based programs.

7. Propose and evaluate policy-based strategies that are likely to improve access to community-based nursing services such as pediatric hospice and nurse practitioner services.

8. Contrast the major economic approaches for evaluating healthcare programs and services.

9. Outline the design for a cost analysis strategy of a healthcare program or service that considers the full costs of society.

10. Analyze pay for performance as a strategy for changing healthcare provider behavior, citing the strengths and weaknesses of this general approach.

11. Identify the potential outcomes as well as unintended consequences that may be expected within pay-for-performance environments.

Managed Care

Managed care is a generic term that can be defined as "a system of health care that combines delivery and payment; and influences utilization of services, by employing management techniques designed to promote the delivery of cost-effective health care" (U.S. Department of Health and Human Services [USDHSS], 2008). With the emergence of a wide range of managed care delivery models over time, the definition of managed care has become less precise. One that may better fit today's version of managed care is "a system of health care delivery that tries to manage the cost of health care, the quality of health care, and access to that care" (Halverson, Kaluzny, & McLaughlin, 1998). In this definition, the concept of integrating the financing and delivery of care is no longer considered a necessary feature to be considered managed care.

During the 1980s, the predominant models of managed care organizations were health maintenance organizations (HMOs) and preferred provider organizations (PPOs). Over time the number of types of managed care organizations (MCOs) grew, and operational distinctions between the models began to blur. This text briefly describes several managed care models prior to presenting cases that elucidate features of these models.

Health maintenance organization (HMO) has been defined as "an entity that provides, offers or arranges for coverage of designated health services needed by members for a fixed, prepaid premium" (USDHSS, 2008). The concept of the prepaid health plan has been omitted from the more general definition that follows: "organized health systems that are responsible for both the financing and the delivery of a broad range of comprehensive health services to an enrolled population" (Kongstvedt, 1994). Traditionally, HMOs are structured as one of three basic models: staff model, group model, and independent practice association (IPA) model (USDHSS, 2008). In the salaried staff model HMO, physicians and other healthcare providers are employed by the HMO (Tufts Managed Care Institute [TMCI], 1998). In the group model, the HMO generally contracts with a single group of healthcare providers to serve the healthcare needs of the enrolled population (TMCI, 1998). And, in the IPA model, the HMO contracts with individual providers of care or an association of individual providers or practices to deliver care to enrolled HMO members (USDHSS, 2008).

Health maintenance organizations typically include features such as contracts between the HMO administrative entity and providers of care with varying types of reimbursement arrangements, a primary care provider acting as a gatekeeper of services, utilization management, quality improvement initiatives, and financial incentives for enrollees to use the contracted providers. Traditionally, within HMOs care was covered when enrollees used contracted providers and not covered when enrollees chose to use noncontracted providers. In some HMOs the providers may assume some level of financial risk, as through a capitation arrangement. Other types of HMOs exist, such as network, direct contract, social, closed panel, and open panel HMOs (TMCI, 1998).

Preferred provider organizations (PPOs) are healthcare systems that typically involve contractual arrangements between a network of próviders and a payer. The providers agree to offer their services to enrolled participants in exchange for certain considerations, such as discounted reimbursement and utilization management controls (Kongstvedt, 1994). The PPO often encourages providers to participate by limiting the number of providers included in the care delivery network(s). The structure of a PPO is similar to the IPA-type HMO. However, in the PPO enrolled participants typically receive coverage for services for both the contracted (in-network) and noncontracted providers. If the enrollee chooses a noncontract provider, the enrollee is likely to be responsible for higher cost sharing, such as higher deductibles, copayments, and/or coinsurance, than if the enrollee chooses to receive care from contracted providers. For example, if the patient uses a contracted (network) provider, the patient may be responsible to pay out-of-pocket expenses at a rate of 10% of the contracted amount. If the patient uses a noncontracted provider, the patient's out-of-pocket personal responsibility might be 30% of charges. Another distinguishing feature of a traditional PPO compared to the HMO is the lack of the gatekeeper concept.

The exclusive provider organization (EPO) is very similar to the PPO managed care structure. Yet, in the EPO, if the enrollee uses an out-of-network healthcare provider, the enrollee must pay for the entire cost of the care (Madlin, 1991). In the EPO system, the health plan does not pay for services that are obtained from noncontract providers. This is similar to what occurs with traditional HMOs. However, in the EPO, as with the PPO, the primary care provider is not responsible to act as a gatekeeper of services.

Point of service (POS) health plans are also referred to as open-ended HMOs (TMCI, 1998). These plans have similar features to the traditional HMO. However, in the POS plan the enrollee has the option of seeking care from nonparticipating providers by paying higher out-of-pocket costs (USDHSS, 2008). For example, if the enrollee obtains services from a contracted primary care provider, the enrollee may be responsible for paying a per-visit copayment of $20. And, if the enrollee seeks care out-of-network, he or she may be responsible for paying, for example, 30% of charges (coinsurance). This plan blends many of the features of HMOs with the patient financial incentive structure generally found in PPOs.

Primary care case management (PCCM) and enhanced primary care case management (E-PCCM) systems are forms of managed care that are used by some state Medicaid programs. These types of managed care systems generally aim to manage the costs and quality of care delivery, but they may not blend the financing and care delivery as might be found with more traditional forms of managed care. In both the PCCM and E-PCCM models of care, primary care providers are expected to provide and coordinate care for their assigned patients. Primary care providers are typically paid a small monthly fee in exchange for coordinating care for their patients. In the E-PCCM model, the PCCM structure is enhanced with other services, as described in the E-PCCM case study. Comparisons of the traditional models of managed care are displayed in **Table 5-1**.

The Uninsured and Access to Healthcare Services

THE UNINSURED: BACKGROUND

In 2006, an estimated 46,995,000 people, or approximately 16% of the U.S. population, had no health insurance (U.S. Census Bureau, 2007). This was an increase of more than 5 million uninsured persons since 2001, a recession year (Center on Budget and Policy Priorities [CBPP], 2006). The decrease in those with health insurance was attributed to the erosion in employer-sponsored health insurance (CBPP, 2006). Often the uninsured were in working families whose employers did not offer health insurance coverage (Kaiser Commission on Medicaid and the Uninsured [KCMU], 2008). More than 70% of the uninsured were in families where at least one person was working full time (KCMU, 2007a). An additional 11% of the uninsured were in families with a part-time worker (KCMU, 2007a). Often the uninsured were self-employed or working for small firms that were less likely to offer health insurance coverage (KCMU, 2007a).

Low-income workers were at greatest risk of being uninsured, with 24.4% of persons with annual incomes less than $25,000 uninsured during 2005 (CBPP, 2006). The majority of uninsured

TABLE 5-1 General Features of Traditional Managed Care Models of Care Delivery

Acronym	HMO	PPO	EPO	POS	PCCM
Name	Health Maintenance Organization	Preferred Provider Organization	Exclusive Provider Organization	Point of Service Plan	Primary Care Case Management
Primary care provider/gatekeeper	Yes	Not typically	Not typically	Yes	Yes
Coverage outside of provider network	Historically 0%	Yes, typically higher enrollee out-of-pocket payments if use out-of-network providers	0%	Yes, typically higher enrollee out-of-pocket payments if use out-of-network providers	May vary
Utilization management (UM)	Referrals to specialists; other UM	Often UM for IP services; may vary for other services	Often UM for IP services; may vary for other services	Referrals, other UM	May vary

Note: IP = inpatient. Models may vary and may be developed as hybrids.

CASE STUDIES

A series of case studies is presented to provide an overview of the operations and features of several distinct managed care models. The first case describes a traditional HMO that is based on the independent practice association (IPA) model. The second case describes a management organization that develops provider networks and systems that support a PPO model. The third case describes a Medicaid managed care program that is structured as an enhanced primary care case management (E-PCCM) model of care delivery. Each case highlights key attributes and goals of managed care systems and several variations that distinguish these models. The first two cases are set in the 1980s at a time when the managed care models were more easily distinguishable. Over time, with the development of many hybrid models, the attributes of various managed care models have become less distinct. However, the case studies demonstrate the goals of these entities and the strategies that have been used to attempt to achieve these goals.

CASE 1: SETTING UP A MEDICAID HEALTH MAINTENANCE ORGANIZATION IN WISCONSIN

BRIEF LEGISLATIVE HISTORY OF MEDICAID

The Social Security Act of 1935 established Aid to Families with Dependent Children (AFDC). This program provided grants to states to supply cash payments to needy children whose families met specific income and other criteria (Social Security Act, Pub. L. 74-271). Title XIX of the Social Security Act established Medicaid in 1965 to pay for healthcare services for persons who were poor or disabled (Wisconsin Department of Health Services [WDHS], 2008). That year, the link between Medicaid health benefit eligibility and receipt of AFDC cash assistance was established by the Social Security Amendments of 1965 (P.L. 89–97) (KCMU, 2001a). Thirty-one years later, AFDC was replaced with Temporary Assistance for Needy Families (TANF) block grants through the Personal Responsibility and Work Opportunity Act of 1996 (PRWOA) (P.L. 104–193). Under TANF, Medicaid was no longer linked with eligibility for cash assistance.

MEDICAID AND MANAGED CARE

Mandatory managed care programs were introduced into Medicaid in the 1980s. The managed care option was made available to states through the Omnibus Reconciliation Act of 1981 (OBRA 81) and section 1915(b), the Managed Care/Freedom of Choice Waivers (KCMU, 2001b). Section 1915(b) allowed states to implement managed care delivery systems or programs that limited provider choice (Centers for Medicare and Medicaid Services [CMS], 2005b). Section 1115 Research and Demonstration Project Waivers also provided states with opportunities to implement statewide managed care programs through comprehensive healthcare reform demonstration programs (KCMU, 2001b).

Wisconsin was one of the first states to implement managed care programs in the AFDC Medicaid population by receiving a federal waiver in the early 1980s (WDHS, 2008). In 1983 the Wisconsin legislature enacted the Medicaid HMO Preferred Enrollment Initiative in response to state fiscal pressures and the desire to contain Medicaid costs (Rowland & Lyons, 1987). This required AFDC recipients living in Milwaukee and Dane Counties to choose an HMO. Wisconsin solicited proposals and bids and then signed contracts with eight HMOs in Milwaukee during the fall of 1983. A ninth HMO was added in Milwaukee County during 1985 (Rowland & Lyons, 1987). More than 100,000 persons were enrolled in Medicaid HMOs in Milwaukee during the first year of operation.

THE OPERATIONS OF ONE MEDICAID HMO IN MILWAUKEE COUNTY

One HMO that served Medicaid recipients in Milwaukee County is described from the perspective of a nurse, the director of operations for the HMO. The HMO in this case study is referred to as NewCare HMO, a fictitious name. NewCare HMO was provider sponsored; it was developed by the umbrella corporation that owned the HMO, hospital, and other related corporate entities. A primary reason that providers, such as hospitals and hospital systems, sponsored and developed HMOs was to help the affiliated hospitals retain their market share of Medicaid business. This retention of market share was possible because HMOs typically contract with or hire a limited number of providers where coverage is available for delivered healthcare services. In the 1980s with the influx of new HMOs to the Milwaukee market, hospitals needed to protect their ability to admit their existing share of Medicaid patients. Developing a Medicaid HMO was one way for hospitals to accomplish this goal through obtaining a contract with the sponsoring HMO.

Each HMO received approximately $65 per member per month (PMPM) from the state during the first contract year. For this amount the HMOs were to provide coverage for all Medicaid services except dental and chiropractic services (Rowland & Lyons, 1987). This monthly capitation rate from the states to the HMOs was expected to result in cost savings for the Wisconsin Medicaid program. However, the capitation rate posed challenges for the HMOs because they needed to expend no more than this capitation payment for healthcare services and administrative expenses to remain financially viable.

The primary activities of NewCare HMO, in the planning and early implementation stages, included negotiating provider contracts and developing a claims processing system, marketing plan, enrollee educational materials, and utilization management and quality improvement programs.

NewCare HMO was structured as an independent practice association (IPA) model. It contracted with a group of providers and specifically targeted those providers who admitted patients to the sponsoring hospital system. Participating primary care providers agreed, under contract, to accept discounted fee-for-service reimbursement from the HMO and to deliver urgent care to their respective primary care enrollees, 24 hours a day, 7 days a week. Contracts were also negotiated with a limited number of hospitals with several goals in mind: (1) contract with the affiliated (sponsoring) hospital to retain Medicaid business; (2) contract with a sufficient number of hospitals to meet the needs of the enrolled population; (3) contract with the only children's hospital in the geographic area to meet the healthcare needs of children; and (4) contain costs through securing discounted reimbursement rates.

Once Medicaid recipients were enrolled with NewCare HMO and had selected primary care providers, one of the greatest challenges faced by the HMO was working to change longstanding care-seeking behavior patterns because many enrollees used emergency departments for primary care services. NewCare HMO developed materials to try to educate enrollees about the concept of a primary care provider (PCP) and the need to work with the PCP to coordinate care. The HMO developed the brochures at approximately a sixth-grade reading level. These were mailed to new enrollees. Educational efforts were supplemented with contract language that required PCPs to provide or contract for services 24 hours a day, 7 days a week. Yet, this contract provision was difficult to monitor and enforce. Additionally, the HMO attempted to deny payments to emergency departments for nonemergent care. However, this approach was quickly disallowed; HMOs needed to reimburse emergency departments even for nonemergent or nonurgent care. Therefore, emergency departments had little or no incentive to work with HMOs to help change enrollee care-seeking behavior patterns. In the early stages of HMO development, the operational systems were deficient, at best, for changing inappropriate utilization.

The director of operations drafted the initial plans for the utilization review and quality management initiatives. These crude systems, initiated prior to extensive use of electronic information systems in the field, included paper copy request forms for inpatient stays and referrals to specialists. A second nurse was then hired as director of utilization review and quality management to lead and develop systems to curb unnecessary spending and enhance quality of care. The director was responsible for establishing guidelines for approval of inpatient stays using best available evidence and existing standards of utilization review. She also reviewed the written requests for inpatient stays. The HMO medical director reviewed denials of hospitalization coverage and denial appeals.

The director of operations wrote the claims processing system specifications using the state's contract as a guide for meeting state reporting expectations. The director worked with university-based programmers to develop a homegrown claims processing system. This system tracked receipt and payment of claims and contracted reimbursement rates. Claims received from specialists that were not accompanied by a completed and signed referral from the PCP were denied payment. Over time these systems were refined.

CASE 2: NETWORK AND SYSTEMS DEVELOPMENT FOR PREFERRED PROVIDER ORGANIZATIONS

The development of provider networks for a preferred provider organization (PPO) is described from the perspective of a nurse who negotiated hospital contracts for this entity. The organization in this case study is referred to as AmeriCare PPO.

AmeriCare PPO established PPO networks and systems in several major metropolitan areas throughout the United States for both commercial health plans and workers' compensation plans. The context for this case study is a multicounty metropolitan area with more than 100 hospitals. The goal was to develop a network of healthcare providers that would serve large corporations with self-funded health plans, workers' compensation programs, and small businesses that were grouped within a business structure for purposes of insuring their employees.

INFORMATION GATHERING PRIOR TO CONTRACT NEGOTIATION ACTIVITIES

The first step in developing a provider network was identifying and collecting information about the hospitals in the geographic service area. The hospital-specific information needed for contracting included size, location, corporate affiliations with other hospitals (e.g., hospital systems), specific types of services provided, volume of specific services, historic costs by type of service, and measures of "quality."

Quality is a difficult concept to measure, even with a large, well-funded research study. Trying to measure quality quickly for purposes of contracting often involves gathering information about the reputation of hospitals from persons in the geographic area and relying on the premise that providers who perform larger volumes of specific services may be more experienced and have better outcomes than those who perform smaller volumes (Birkmeyer et al., 2003).

In addition, it was important to examine past hospital utilization patterns of clients to be served by the networks to determine which hospitals were important to include in a network to acknowledge preferences of the customers to be served. It was believed that the system would be most successful if existing utilization patterns were supported in the network contracting process.

Another step in the data collection process involved plotting all of the hospital locations and names on a map of the service area. Next, using information gathered from key informants, small geographic service areas including approximately four to six hospitals that may have been in direct competition with each other were identified and plotted on the map. Hospitals within each small geographic area were then ranked to determine the desired target hospitals to contract with.

CONTRACT NEGOTIATIONS WITH CARE PROVIDERS

AmeriCare PPO began the contracting process by sending packets of information to all hospitals in the service area, asking them to bid to participate. The packets included a standard managed care contract with provisions that reflected the operational goals of AmeriCare PPO. The packets also included a bid sheet asking the providers to list proposed per diem reimbursement rates for medical, surgical, obstetric, and other types of inpatient services; percentage discounts with caps for outpatient services; and per case rates for some very expensive services such as transplants and open heart surgeries. AmeriCare negotiators followed up on the mailed solicitations with phone calls.

In some service areas the contracting process involved convincing hospitals to participate in the bidding and/or contract negotiation process. Those hospitals with seemingly few competitors or with very high occupancy or with a low risk of losing significant market share were more difficult to convince to enter the bidding process. The process of convincing target hospitals to bid, participate in the program, agree to contract terms, and offer the best reimbursement rates was complex.

Negotiation approaches were based on "win-win" principles (Ury & Fisher, 1988). The process involved talking with hospital administrators by phone or preferably in person and listening to determine what was important to the hospital. For example, some providers were interested in increasing their inpatient volume, decreasing administrative burdens associated with some healthcare plans, and having claims paid promptly. AmeriCare PPO worked to meet some of the needs of providers in exchange for favorable (discounted) reimbursement rates. For example, by contracting with only about 20% to 25% of hospitals in a geographic area, it was expected that in-network hospitals would gain some new business that currently went to competing out-of-network hospitals. New business, even if discounted new business, can be helpful to hospitals by covering some of their fixed or overhead costs, such as for the facility and utilities.

To channel enrollees to in-network providers it was believed that at least a 20 percentage point differential needed to exist between the in-network and out-of-network coinsurance levels. For example, if patients are to pay 20% of the inpatient bill when they use a network provider versus 40% of the bill when they use an out-of-network (noncontracted) provider, it is believed that most patients will choose to receive care from the in-network providers. If patients use the in-network providers, AmeriCare PPO would pay for care at the discounted/contracted rate, and the patient would be expected to pay fewer out-of-pocket costs. By using in-network providers, not only do patients pay the smaller coinsurance percentage but they also pay coinsurance on a smaller amount, on the contracted reimbursement amount rather than a percentage of full charges. Channeling patients to in-network providers within workers' compensation plans was more complicated in states that did not permit provider choice restrictions. In those states the channeling process involved educating the workplace benefits managers and encouraging these managers to persuade injured or sick employees to use contracted providers (Resnick, 1992).

After the hospital provider network had been established within AmeriCare PPO, the process of contracting with primary care and specialty care providers began. In general, AmeriCare PPO focused on contracting with providers who had admitting privileges or worked at the contracted hospitals. For example, contracts needed to be negotiated with anesthesiology, radiology, pathology, and emergency department care providers who billed separately from the contracted hospitals. Negotiating contracts with hospital-based care providers after hospital contracts had been negotiated proved challenging because these providers often did not believe they needed to offer discounted care to maintain their market share of clients. Because of their relationship with the hospital they would receive the business even if they refused to contract with AmeriCare PPO.

UTILIZATION MANAGEMENT INITIATIVES

A second approach to cost containment in AmeriCare PPO was utilization management (UM). The primary strategy used was a concurrent review process of inpatient hospital stays. When AmeriCare PPO patients were hospitalized the network provider had the contractual responsibility to notify the designated contracted utilization management firm with the hospitalization details. The UM firm sent nurse reviewers to the hospitals to monitor hospitalizations. The concurrent review process involved medical record review by a nurse reviewer to determine, using established criteria, whether the inpatient stay seemed appropriate. The nurse returned to the hospital to review records periodically to determine whether inpatient care continued to be required.

The intervals between medical record reviews were individualized based on the needs and health conditions of each admitted patient. If inpatient care did not seem appropriate, the hospital was given notice that the patient should be discharged within a specific period of time (e.g., within 24 hours). Reimbursement for care would occur up to the specified time period. An appeals process could be initiated when the providers believed that patients required longer inpatient stays. The use of second surgical opinions was another UM approach used with the intent of reducing unnecessary care.

PROCESS IMPROVEMENT ACTIVITIES

AmeriCare PPO implemented a system for documenting, addressing, and monitoring questions, concerns, and complaints. This system was very simple yet operationally structured to ensure all issues that came to the attention of the organization were handled. The nurse contract negotiator hired a full-time customer services employee whose primary responsibility was to answer any questions, by phone, from patients, providers, or the public. The customer service representative reported directly to the nurse contract negotiator. This reporting relationship facilitated communication about important issues that might affect future or existing contracts. In addition, the contract negotiator's detailed knowledge of the contract provisions was often critical for helping to resolve questions and concerns.

The customer service employee documented every phone call on a one-page hard-copy form. Each case remained open until fully resolved. The customer service representative reviewed challenging cases with the contract negotiator on a regular basis, often several times per day. Key elements of each case, such as the type of question or complaint, were entered into a computerized tracking system for reporting purposes. Summary reports from this data system were used to identify trends in questions, concerns, and complaints. These trends were then used to plan systems improvements. This system for process improvement was successful, in part, because the system centered on documentation and follow-up. However, the diligence and customer service approach of the individual employees contributed substantially to the success of this system.

CASE 3: ENHANCED PRIMARY CARE CASE MANAGEMENT MODEL FOR MEDICAID RECIPIENTS

Throughout the 1980s and 1990s, state Medicaid programs increasingly shifted Medicaid enrollment into managed care models with the intent of increasing access to care and slowing expenditure growth (Fleisher, 2003; Holahan & Suzuki, 2003; Landon, Huskamp, Tobias, & Epstein, 2000; Miller & Gengler, 1993; Smith, Cotter, McClish, Bovbjerg, & Rossiter, 2000; Smith, Cotter, & Rossiter, 1996; Sofaer, Woolley, Kenney, Kreling, & Mauery, 1998). The Medicaid managed care programs vary from state to state in terms of administrative structure, implementation and enrollment guidelines, program elements, payment methods, and regulatory environments (Brodsky & Baron, 2000; Cooper & Kuhlthau, 2001).

One managed care model, primary care case management (PCCM), was first introduced into Medicaid in Michigan and Utah in 1982 and 1983, respectively (Highsmith & Somers, 2000; Hurley & Draper, 2002; Zuckerman, Brennan, & Yemane, 2002). Within the PCCM model of care, Medicaid enrollees are linked with primary care providers who act as gatekeepers of services, provide medical homes, and coordinate care (Rawlings-Sekunda, Curtis, & Kaye, 2001; Schulman, Sheriff, & Momany, 1997). Primary care providers, in most state PCCM Medicaid programs, are paid on a fee-for-service (FFS) basis and receive nominal monthly management fees for assigned or self-selected Medicaid recipients (Adams, Bronstein, & Florence, 2003; Schneider, Landon, Tobias, & Epstein, 2004; Schoenman, Evans, & Schur, 1997). Primary care case management programs are generally designed with the intent of increasing beneficiary use of primary and preventive care in primary care provider offices; decreasing use of specialty and urgent care; improving timeliness, quality, and continuity of care; and decreasing overall costs (Adams et al., 2003; Dallek, Parks, & Waxman, 1984; Muller & Baker, 1996).

In North Carolina, the Medicaid program evolved from traditional fee-for-service to primary care case management (PCCM) models in 1991. In 1998, the North Carolina Medicaid program initiated a unique and innovative approach to managed care called Community Care of North Carolina (CCNC). This program is structured as a PCCM model that is enhanced with special services such as local case management, disease management services, and quality improvement initiatives. This managed care structure is often referred to as enhanced primary care case management (E-PCCM). Within CCNC there are 14 distinct networks that work collaboratively with the state of North Carolina to manage the care of Medicaid recipients (Community Care of North Carolina, 2008). The largest network began as a statewide group of primary care providers. Some networks are structured as partnerships established within specific geographic regions such as a group of counties. The networks are responsible for actually managing the care delivery by emphasizing the primary care provider as a coordinator of care and through special services provided by case managers.

Community-based case management services combined with a population-based approach to health services delivery are features critical to managing care within CCNC. Primarily, community-based case managers are registered nurses, social workers, and health educators. They are responsible for assessing the health, functional abilities, and psychosocial needs of clients; coordinating care with community service agencies and other care providers; educating clients about health and health behaviors; supporting clients through lifestyle changes; and monitoring health status and care delivery. Case managers are often assigned to one or more primary care practices. They may be based out of a specific practice or an alternate location. This process may vary from network to network. The case managers may each be assigned to a population of approximately 2,500 enrollees; some case managers who serve pediatric populations may have higher caseloads. Yet, within these caseloads the case managers primarily focus on specific patients who are identified as having specific needs for case coordination.

Electronic data systems support the population-based strategies within CCNC. Case managers use a customized web-based clinical information system to identify clients who may need services and to document coordination of care, plans, interventions, and outcomes. The clinical information system is also used to track disease management activities.

Two nursing challenges faced in the E-PCCM environment are supervising case managers and demonstrating effectiveness and cost-effectiveness of case management and disease management services. Because case managers in some networks are distributed throughout the state, supervision of activities often relies on the use of standardized electronic reports and review of documentation rather than on direct supervision. Limitations of data systems can compromise monitoring and supervision. In addition, case managers may have dual reporting relationships when both the clinical practice and the central network administration are responsible for directing case management activities. At times the needs of the clinical practice may conflict with and supersede the goals of the overall program. Evaluation of case management services often poses additional challenges. First, in many programs specific evaluation plans were not developed during program planning phases, making evaluation data potentially less accessible. Data collection plans also tend to focus on the needs of the care coordinators and care providers rather than on the needs of those evaluating programs. Second, the diversity of case management services and variations between networks and case managers can lead to measurement challenges (Boult, Rassen, Rassen, Moore, & Robison, 2000). Third, case management services often operate within complex healthcare delivery systems and diverse environments and cultures. Therefore, it can be challenging to isolate the effects of case management from other services and influences (Jacobson Vann, 2006).

DISCUSSION QUESTIONS:

1. Describe at least three goals of managed care organizations. Discuss and critique the mechanisms that may be used to achieve these goals. Contrast the implied goals of the different types of managed care models of care delivery.

2. Develop a brief plan describing how advanced practice nurses (APNs) can position themselves to provide services to managed care enrollees. Discuss the services or unique approaches that APNs can potentially offer managed care organizations to make contracting a win-win situation.

3. When contemplating a win-win contract with a managed care organization, what would you, as an APN, expect from the contract in exchange for discounted reimbursement?

4. Develop a plan that describes the types of operational systems that APNs should develop or enhance to serve a managed care population.

5. Analyze the three managed care case studies and describe recurrent themes (goals, attributes) that are common to the systems of care delivery. Also, distinguish attributes and goals that are different among them.

6. Identify the type of managed care structure that you would prefer to participate in as a contracted provider. Describe at least two reasons why this system of managed care is preferable to you.

7. Analyze the emphasis on quality of care within each of the three models of managed care delivery as described in the case studies. Provide rationales for your answer.

persons were not eligible for public programs, yet could not afford coverage without financial assistance (KCMU, 2007b). African Americans (19.6%) and Hispanics (32.7%) were more likely to be uninsured than were white, non-Hispanics (11.3%) (CBPP, 2006).

The uninsured were less likely to seek healthcare services, receive preventive services, and have a regular care provider than were those who had health insurance (KCMU, 2007a; Mauksch et al., 2003). In 2005, uninsured women who participated in the National Health Interview Survey reported the lowest use (38.3%) of mammography screening services (Sabatino et al., 2008).

For the estimated 11 million uninsured persons with chronic illnesses, the negative access-to-care trends were also evident, based on results from the National Health and Nutrition Examination Survey (1999–2004). Uninsured persons with chronic illnesses were less likely to visit a healthcare professional, less likely to have a usual site for care, and more likely to use the emergency department for care than were insured persons with chronic illnesses (Wilper et al., 2008). The consequences of being uninsured and not seeking care early included excess deaths and poorer health outcomes (KCMU, 2007a; Wilper et al., 2008).

BREAST AND CERVICAL CANCER LEGISLATION

Breast and Cervical Cancer Mortality Prevention Act of 1990

Women who are underserved, uninsured, or underinsured may qualify for free or low-cost breast or cervical cancer screening tests through the Centers for Disease Control and Prevention's National Breast and Cervical Cancer Early Detection Program (Centers for Disease Control and Prevention [CDC], 2007). This program was established by the Breast and Cervical Cancer Mortality Prevention Act of 1990 (P.L. 101–354) (CDC, 2007). It operates in all 50 states, the District of Columbia, many U.S. territories, and 12 American Indian/Alaska Native organizations (CDC, 2007). The general eligibility guidelines include those uninsured and underinsured women at or below 250% of the federal poverty level (FPL) and those women of screening age (CDC, 2008). For a family of two in 2008, 250% of the FPL was $35,000 in most states (USDHHS, 2008). Women can locate programs and determine whether they are eligible for services by checking the Centers for Disease Control and Prevention (CDC) website, which lists contact information for each state, territory, and American Indian/Alaskan Native organization (CDC, 2008).

Breast and Cervical Cancer Prevention and Treatment Act

In October 2000, under the Clinton administration, Congress passed the Breast and Cervical Cancer Prevention and Treatment

Act to supplement the efforts of the Breast and Cervical Cancer Mortality Prevention Act of 1990 (CMS, 2005a). This act provides states with the opportunity to expand Medicaid coverage to women in need of treatment for breast and cervical cancer as a Medicaid optional eligibility category. Women may be eligible for Medicaid coverage under this category if they are: (1) screened through the National Breast and Cervical Cancer Early Detection Program (NBCCEDP) and are found to have breast or cervical cancer; (2) under 65 years of age; and (3) uninsured and not eligible for Medicaid under other eligibility categories (CMS, 2005a).

CASE STUDY: *The Uninsured*

This case study highlights the challenges faced by those in the United States who lack health insurance coverage.

A 53-year-old woman presents in Plum Clinic during August for a checkup. The woman, referred to as Eliza, complains of a breast lump that she had noticed a while back. She delayed getting this lump checked because she lacked health insurance coverage. Eliza is well-educated, with bachelor's and master's degrees in art. She is employed, yet cannot afford health insurance because the premium cost would be approximately 50% of her current income. She previously lost health insurance coverage when her employer downsized the art department. Her husband also works as an artist and educator. Their combined income is less than 250% of the federal poverty level. Eliza and her husband live in a rural area and raise and grow organic food for their own consumption. Eliza had read about a free breast cancer screening program previously, yet was unable to find information about this program when she noticed the lump. She does not have Internet access at home and must go to the local library to use the Internet.

During Eliza's health history, she complained that her neighbors, who farm, have pesticides applied to their fields using crop dusting techniques. She is concerned that this toxic exposure may have contributed to the development of her breast lump. In addition, Eliza lives in southwestern Minnesota, an area known for relatively high levels of arsenic in ground water and wells (Minnesota Pollution Control Agency, 1998).

Prior to receiving any diagnostic procedures or other care, Eliza alerted the clinicians and clerical staff at each healthcare facility she visited that she was uninsured. In all her encounters with healthcare providers, none provided her with written or verbal information about the SAGE program, Minnesota's Breast and Cervical Cancer Early Detection Program. After Eliza received a physical examination, her primary care provider referred her for a mammogram at a local healthcare center that had previously been a SAGE provider. The mammogram showed abnormal results. Eliza was referred immediately to a surgeon for a biopsy and then a mastectomy. Prior to the mastectomy Eliza inquired about the costs of services. She was reassured that the hospital had a policy to bill uninsured persons at a discounted rate and was informed that the cost of all physician services would be included in the cost of hospital care.

Eliza later received a hospital bill exceeding $9,000 and separate physician bills totaling more than $6,000. The team of healthcare providers recommended that Eliza receive chemotherapy. However, Eliza refused further treatment because of a lack of health insurance coverage.

DISCUSSION QUESTIONS:

1. What seems to have gone wrong with Eliza's care at the point of entry into the "healthcare" delivery system?

2. Knowing that Eliza does not have health insurance coverage, what approaches would you, as a nurse or advanced practice nurse, suggest to help her access necessary care for screening and treatment of the breast cancer (1) at the point of initial contact when she came in for a physical exam, and (2) after she had the mastectomy?

3. What federal and/or state policy changes would you recommend to improve health access in cases such as this? Describe three specific recommendations.

4. Analyze the Centers for Disease Control and Prevention's National Breast and Cervical Cancer Early Detection Program and the Breast and Cervical Cancer Prevention and Treatment Act of 2000. Outline the pros and cons of these laws. Describe at least one change that you would propose to improve access to care.

Funding Strategies for Nurse-Managed Health Centers and Other Community-Based Services

Nurse-managed health centers are managed and staffed by registered nurses and advanced practice nurses, such as nurse practitioners (Torrisi & Hansen-Turton, 2005). These centers are based in the community and often serve vulnerable and underserved populations (National Nursing Centers Consortium, 2014). The care delivered in nurse-managed centers generally follows the holistic model and focuses not only on treating problems but on promoting health. Despite the benefits offered by these centers to those who may not otherwise have access to healthcare services, these innovative models of care delivery often face barriers with respect to obtaining funding from traditional sources of reimbursement (Torrisi & Hansen-Turton, 2005).

The cases in this section describe examples of innovative programs, including a pediatric hospice, a nurse-managed health center, and a prevention-focused cardiology clinic, to highlight some of the challenges these organizations face in obtaining funding and remaining viable.

Fee-for-service Medicaid programs are required to cover services provided by some advanced practice nurses, such as pediatric nurse practitioners, family nurse practitioners, and certified nurse–midwives (American Nurses Association [ANA], 2008). States have the option to cover the services of other types of advanced practice nurses. Within Medicaid managed care programs, including primary care case management delivery systems, states have the option to include or exclude nurse practitioners from participating as providers and as primary care case managers (ANA, 2008). The states make the decisions regarding reimbursement rates for advanced practice nurses for Medicaid programs.

In 1997 Congress authorized nurse practitioners to be directly reimbursed for care provided to patients covered by Medicare (Buppert, 2004). The specific rules and reimbursement guidelines are not outlined here. However, the implications of Medicare reimbursement of nurse practitioner services include not only the direct and obvious benefits but the indirect benefits of helping to open the doors for other third-party payers to follow Medicare's lead.

CASE STUDIES

CASE 1: EDMARC HOSPICE FOR CHILDREN

Edmarc Hospice for Children was established in 1978 as the first hospice designed specifically for children in the United States. Its mission is to "ease the trauma of a child's illness or death, and to reduce the disabling effects of pediatric illness, loss, and bereavement on families" (Edmarc Hospice for Children, 2008). This program was founded by members of the Suffolk Presbyterian Church in Suffolk, Virginia; the minister of the church, who was dying of cancer; and the parents of a young boy who was dying of a progressive neuromuscular disease. The parents of the young boy searched for services within the healthcare industry to allow their son to receive care at home. Given the lack of available services, this family turned to their church for assistance. The hospice was named in memory of the minister, Edward, and the boy, Marcus.

Edmarc Hospice is licensed as a hospice and is certified as a home care agency. Edmarc provides holistic care that focuses on the needs of children and their families. Its programs and services span home health and hospice care, patient and family support, and bereavement support. The services are structured to allow children to stay in the comfort of their own homes with their families as much as possible. Home health and hospice care services are delivered by registered nurses and are directed by physicians. Nursing care is available to patients and families 24 hours a day, 7 days a week. Medical social workers provide individual and group support to parents, patients, and siblings. When families experience the loss of a child, Edmarc provides one-on-one support through home visits, telephone calls, and educational materials. In addition, Edmarc sponsors family events throughout the year, such as an Easter Egg Hunt, family picnic, and Halloween party. Edmarc relies heavily on a wide range of volunteers, such as the medical director, assistant medical director, Spanish interpreter, and many others. The Peace by Piece community outreach and peer support program is staffed by volunteer facilitators who go through a rigorous training program.

Edmarc, incorporated in 1978, got its start as a volunteer organization. In 1982 a nurse executive from a local healthcare organization assisted the Edmarc board of directors with preparing a grant proposal to be submitted to Presbyterian Women, the national women's organization of the Presbyterian Church. The proposal was funded, and Edmarc received a $300,000 grant (Edmarc Hospice for Children, 2008). This initial seed money enabled the agency to expand, hire employees, and continue with its mission of helping children with life-threatening illnesses as well as their families.

In fiscal year 2008, the annual operating budget was approximately $900,000. Only about 10% of this amount came from third-party reimbursement for services, from payers such as Tricare, Medicaid, and private insurance companies. Edmarc bills third-party payers for authorized visits, generally only those visits made by registered nurses. However, a few third-party payers authorize payment for visits made by medical social workers. Reimbursement amounts vary by payer and range from approximately 30% to 80% of charges. Families are not balance-billed for unpaid services. An estimated 90% of funding comes from charitable contributions, fund-raising events, grants, and other sources. During 2007, an endowment campaign was launched with the goal of raising $5 million. These funds were needed to enhance clinical care by increasing the number of nursing staff and social workers who providing in-home hospice care, increase bereavement outreach, and create a growth capital fund for the future.

In September 2008, a congressman from Virginia, Jim Moran, introduced legislation that was intended to improve care for children with life-threatening illnesses (Moran, 2008). The Children's Program of All-inclusive, Coordinated Care Act of 2008, or ChiPACC Act (H.R. 6931), allows states the option to provide continuous, coordinated care in the home for children who are seriously ill and enrolled in Medicaid. This act improved upon the existing model of care for these children. Traditionally, children could receive hospice services only if their physician gave them a prognosis of no more than 6 months to live. However, some children vacillate in and out of terminal phases and require both treatment-based and hospice-based services. This legislation allowed children to receive combinations of medical, counseling, respite, and other needed services.

In June 2005, Florida received approval for a federal 1915(b) Medicaid waiver to implement a program based on the ChiPACC model. This 2-year waiver allows the Florida Medicaid program to waive Medicaid hospice laws that prohibit children from receiving hospice services while obtaining curative care (Children's Hospice International, 2008). This waiver also expands coverage for supportive services. Several other states are working on similar programs (Children's Hospice International, 2008).

CASE 2: ENGELHARD MEDICAL CENTER

Engelhard Medical Center is located in Hyde County, North Carolina. In 2007, this rural coastal county had an estimated population of 5,447 (Office of State Budget and Management, 2008). Hyde County covers 613 square miles and has a population density of approximately 10 people per square mile (City-Data.com, 2008). The county has been described as flat with large farms that grow crops such as corn, cotton, soybeans, and broccoli. The closest alternative medical center is estimated to be at least 50 miles away.

Engelhard Medical Center got its start in 2004 at a time when the village of Engelhard's physician of approximately 50 years prepared to retire. The community leaders of Engelhard initiated discussions with healthcare leaders at Eastern Carolina University and the North Carolina Office of Rural Health and Community Care. In one of the local health planning meetings, the retiring physician suggested having the community's health needs met by a nurse practitioner or physician assistant, with backup provided by a physician in relatively close proximity to Engelhard. The program moved forward, and Engelhard Medical Center contracted for services with a nurse practitioner (NP) from a distant county. Weekly, the NP drives a significant distance from her home to provide care to those in need, staying in Engelhard during the week and returning to her home on weekends. The medical center serves about 22 patients per day.

During part of the first year of operation, Engelhard Medical Center was a satellite office of a physician who practices in another town. Before the end of the first year, the board of directors determined that it would be advantageous to split from the physician's office and incorporate as a nonprofit 501(c)3 organization. The NP negotiated a locum tenens contract and is reimbursed by the center on a per diem basis. The clinic operates in a double-wide trailer.

Approximately 80% of funding for clinic operations comes from revenue generated by billed services. Medicare, Medicaid, and Blue Cross/Blue Shield are major payers. One large private insurance company will not certify the NP as a healthcare provider even though she is the only healthcare provider in the county. Some payers require that a physician's name appears on the claims for services delivered by the NP. Uninsured patients may pay for services based on a sliding fee scale. The state of North Carolina provides approximately 20% of medical center funding.

The Rural Health Clinic Services Act (RHC Act) of 1977 was passed to address the problem of an inadequate supply of physicians serving Medicare and Medicaid patients in rural areas. At the time, services provided by midlevel practitioners, such as nurse practitioners and physician assistants, generally were not reimbursed by Medicare and Medicaid. The RHC Act authorized Medicare and Medicaid reimbursement for services provided by midlevel practitioners in designated rural health clinics (USDHHS, Office of Inspector General, 2005). If the Engelhard Medical Center were to receive a Rural Health Clinic designation, it would be eligible to receive enhanced Medicare and Medicaid reimbursement (USDHHS, Office of Inspector General, 2005).

Engelhard Medical Center plans to move its operations out of the double-wide trailer and into a new building when construction is completed. The board discussed the need for a new medical center building because of anticipated growth in the area and the possible development of a marina. A person in the community sold 4 acres of land to the center at a reasonable price to support this effort. The North Carolina Office of Rural Health provided significant support for the real estate purchase. The NP and others involved with the center wrote grant proposals to three foundations and charitable trusts and received grants totaling more than $1 million for the building fund. So far, the community has raised approximately $20,000 of a goal of $50,000.

This medical center is incredibly important to the citizens of this underserved area. County residents highly value the NP and the center. In fact, at the grand opening of the clinic approximately 4,000 people—almost the community's total population—showed up for the celebration.

CASE 3: CARDIOLOGY SPECIALISTS OF THE CAROLINAS

Cardiology Specialists of the Carolinas is an innovative cardiology clinic that is staffed by a team comprising one nurse practitioner and two cardiologists. The practice has been operational in its metropolitan location for 4 weeks and sees patients from 8:15 a.m. to 6:30 p.m., Monday through Friday. In general, a new patient is scheduled to see whichever provider has the next available opening that is convenient to the patient. However, some patients with specific health issues may be scheduled to see the provider specializing in that specific issue. For example, the NP may work with patients who experience erectile dysfunction related to a cardiac problem.

The cardiology team works with patients who have previously had cardiac events as well as those with or without a family history of cardiac problems who are interested in preventing future health problems. The team emphasizes primary, secondary, and tertiary prevention. The typical initial visit at this clinic lasts 1 to 2 hours. During this time, the patients are screened for family, social, lifestyle, work, and exercise history; receive extensive lab and other specialized testing; and discuss plans of care. If patients express readiness to make positive health behavior changes, goals are mutually established, behavior changes are encouraged, and patients are often referred to programs to assist them with meeting their goals. Care providers encourage patients to engage in some type of appropriate physical activity (movement), such as yoga, swimming, or dance, 7 days a week. Examples of referral programs and services include hypnotism for smoking cessation, physical activity programs, and eating disorder programs that support patients who are trying to achieve normal weight. If patients are not ready to make changes, the providers discuss the health risks of continued behaviors.

The practice is structured as a professional corporation. It is owned equally by the three providers. To get started the corporation developed a model of care delivery and a business plan. The group went to a bank familiar with the group's plans and obtained a drawdown loan that allows the practice to withdraw money as needed. According to the NP, the successful development of this program can be attributed, in part, to having a strong, trusted business leader who understands the world of healthcare financial management. In addition, the assistance of a good, reasonable attorney was needed to assist with legal issues. Then, after getting started, the team realized that it takes perseverance, willingness to compromise, and acceptance that some things related to the business side of health care are out of a provider's control.

The clinicians are credentialed by the same third-party payers they had worked with prior to the development of the new corporation. Billing and reimbursement have not been problems, to date. Some payers, such as Medicare Part B, reimburse advanced practice nurses who bill under their own identification numbers 85% of the physician reimbursement amount. The practice has contracted with managed care organizations to provide services to their enrollees.

DISCUSSION QUESTIONS:

1. Design a global funding strategy for pediatric palliative care and nurse-managed health clinics that addresses and facilitates the following issues:

   - Access to necessary services

   - Healthcare cost containment

   - Minimized opportunities for fraud and abuse

   - Existence within the current U.S. healthcare delivery system and legal and political environments

2. Consider who should fund these services and what type of reimbursement structure might support these goals.

Cost Analysis of Healthcare Programs and Services

Since 1940, the rates of increase in healthcare expenditures in the United States have exceeded increases in the GDP (Williams & Torrens, 2002). The United States spends more per capita on healthcare services than any other country (Commonwealth Fund Commission on a High Performance Health System, 2008). In fact, in 2002, U.S. per capita healthcare spending exceeded that of the next highest Organisation for Economic Co-operation and Development (OECD) country, Switzerland, by more than 50% (White, 2007).

Despite the high health and sick care expenditures, U.S. healthcare systems have been ranked comparatively low on performance measures, such as inappropriateness of care, wastefulness, fragmentation, avoidable hospitalizations, and other measures of quality (Commonwealth Fund Commission on a High Performance Health System, 2008). This combination of high levels of healthcare expenditures and relative failure to improve the health status of populations to a commensurate degree demonstrates the need to refocus healthcare delivery systems. Healthcare systems need to shift directions and focus on delivering services that lead to improved health in a cost-effective way. Advanced practice nurses and nurses with management or policymaking responsibility must have the skills to evaluate the outcomes and costs of services to help set new priorities and better utilize scarce healthcare resources in the United States.

COST ANALYSIS APPROACHES

This case study describes several basic concepts related to cost analysis. This description is not intended to outline the complete process of performing cost analyses because the methods can be complex and extensive. Rather, this case provides an overview of general concepts.

The costs of healthcare programs are evaluated using several different approaches. The basic types of economic analyses include cost-benefit analysis, cost-effectiveness analysis, and cost-utility analysis (Drummond, Stoddart, & Torrance, 1989). In all three basic approaches, the costs of the programs or services are estimated the same way. The three approaches differ in how consequences are measured. In cost-benefit analysis, the consequences of programs or services are evaluated in financial terms. In cost-effectiveness analysis, the consequences or outcomes of programs or services are measured in physical units, such as years of life gained (Drummond et al., 1989). And, in cost-utility analysis, the consequences are measured in time units that are adjusted for the quality of the healthcare outcome. Examples of cost-utility measures include quality-adjusted life years (QALYs) and disability-adjusted life years (DALYs) (Vanhook, 2007).

The cost estimation process begins with specifying the evaluation question. The question should be well formulated and include the programs or services to be evaluated and/or compared and the viewpoint or perspective for making comparisons. For example, a state health planning agency may want to compare the relative costs of programs and services needed to prevent childhood obesity with the costs of treating obesity and all of the chronic health problems associated with obesity. If the viewpoint is that of one state Medicaid program, then the evaluation may focus only on the reimbursement amounts that Medicaid is responsible for paying in the short term and long term. If the viewpoint is a societal perspective, then the costs to be enumerated would likely include the direct and indirect costs of care, costs to the patient and family, and costs to society. Costs to the patient and family include items such as time and transportation expenses. Costs to society may include items such as lost productivity, environmental degradation from the delivery of healthcare services, and related costs of treating diseases and disabilities resulting from the environmental impact of healthcare delivery. The expansion of the traditional cost analysis approaches to include societal costs of environmental damage and subsequent adverse health effects may be supported or explained by either complexity economics or ecological economics (Bengston, 1993; Tainter, 1996).

The concept of complexity economics may apply to the U.S. healthcare system because the delivery systems and approaches to care have evolved to be extremely complex within a complex society. The effects of healthcare delivery systems yield both costs and benefits. The benefits to society may include improved health for some and employment for a wide range of health professionals. Yet, the costs of these complex systems can be profound. Hospital-acquired infections and other healthcare errors are costly, both financially and in terms of human costs. In addition, medical waste and pollution result in extensive costs to society in terms of environmental and human health. As the level of complexity in health care has increased, the benefits of this complexity have increased to a point; as complexity continues to increase, the benefits have failed to keep up and in fact may be declining (Tainter, 1996). The health status of U.S. populations lags far behind the health of populations in other developed countries that spend significantly less on healthcare delivery. And the environmental costs of care delivery are great.

Ecological economics addresses the relationships between ecosystems and economic systems (Bengston, 1993). Human activities, such as healthcare delivery, operate on a finite planet. Within the ecological economic framework, it is believed that "the integrity and sustainability of the ecosystem are essential to future economic well-being, and that the criterion of sustainability should be built into economic models and policies" (Bengston, 1993). It then follows that the negative environmental impact of healthcare delivery should be built into cost analyses of healthcare programs and services.

Very rarely are the costs of environmental damage and subsequent health-related injuries, illnesses, and disabilities included in cost analyses of healthcare services. Yet, the financial and health costs associated with environmental pollution and waste are substantial. Hospitals and other healthcare organizations are large contributors to environmental contamination and waste (iatrogenic pollution), and they therefore also contribute to the development and/or aggravation of acute and chronic health problems. Hospitals in the United States generate more than 6,600 tons of waste per day (Shaner-McRae, McRae, & Jas, 2007). This is approximately 1% of all waste produced in the United States. Incineration of waste is a leading source of highly toxic dioxin, mercury, lead, and other dangerous air pollutants (Ferri, 2007). Pharmaceutical waste contaminates the surface, ground, and drinking water (Practice Greenhealth, 2008). This waste is generated through intravenous preparation, compounding, spills, partially used vials or other containers, patients' personal medications, outdated pharmaceuticals, and other sources (Practice Greenhealth, 2008). The energy consumed by healthcare organizations also contributes adversely to health. For example, one study, sponsored by the Maryland Nurses Association, estimated that pollution from six of Maryland's largest coal-burning power plants contributed to 700 deaths per year (Williamson, 2006).

The American Nurses Association's Principles of Environmental Health for Nursing Practice guides environmentally safe nursing care and supports the need to consider the adverse impact of healthcare services on environmental health when performing cost evaluations (ANA, 2007). For example, "the Precautionary Principle guides nurses in their practice to use products and practices that do not harm human health or the environment and to take preventive action in the face of uncertainty" (ANA, 2007, p. 16). The principle of doing no harm may be challenging to achieve in a healthcare system that is heavily treatment focused. However, to the degree that this principle is not achieved, the societal costs of iatrogenic pollution should be accounted for in any cost analysis of healthcare programs and services.

CASE STUDY: *Cost Analysis*

A direct cost analysis was conducted in a group of infants who were born at 32 to 35 weeks estimated gestational age (EGA) during their first year of life (Wegner et al., 2004). These infants were enrolled in the North Carolina Medicaid program and were studied during the 2002 to 2003 respiratory syncytial virus (RSV) season. This study was performed to determine whether the direct costs of palivizumab use to the North Carolina Medicaid program outweighed the costs of treatment associated with serious RSV infection. The costs of RSV-related prophylaxis and treatment were compared between a group of infants who received palivizumab (n = 185) and a group of infants who did not receive prophylaxis (n = 182).

Medicaid claims were obtained for all study participants for the study period. Inpatient claims were reviewed to identify those with prespecified diagnoses. In addition, medical records were abstracted to determine dates of palivizumab administration and results of RSV testing. The average seasonal costs of RSV treatment and prophylaxis were computed for inpatient services, ambulatory care services, emergency department services, palivizumab injections, and total costs (Wegner et al., 2004).

Five children in the prophylaxis (palivizumab) group were hospitalized with an RSV infection or bronchiolitis during the study period compared with 12 children in the comparison group (Wegner et al., 2004). The average drug cost of one palivizumab injection was more than $1,200. With children generally receiving up to five injections during the study period, the average palivizumab drug cost per person in the prophylaxis group was $4,996.46. The average seasonal costs of treatment and prophylaxis in the prophylaxis group were $5,434.20 compared with $504.79 in the nonprophylaxis group. The net cost of prophylaxis to prevent one RSV hospitalization was estimated to be more than $100,000. From the perspective of Medicaid, the direct costs of prophylaxis in infants born at 32 to 35 weeks EGA far outweighed the direct costs of treatment for RSV bronchiolitis.

This cost analysis considered only the direct costs of care to the Medicaid program. If this cost analysis were expanded to consider the costs to the family, the additional items to be enumerated may include items such as those shown in **Table 5-2**.

TABLE 5-2 Examples of Family-Related Costs in a Cost Analysis of Palivizumab Prophylaxis in Children Born at 32 to 35 Weeks EGA, from a Society Perspective

Prophylaxis Group	Comparison (Nonprophylaxis) Group
Up to 5 office visits for palivizumab injections: • Parent time for clinic visits and travel • Cost of travel • Lost time at work and possibly lost income Hospitalization for RSV bronchiolitis:[a] • Parent time for hospital admission and visits • Cost of travel • Lost time at work and possibly lost income and reduced job security Child discomfort: • Injections • RSV-related illnesses that are not prevented	Hospitalization for RSV bronchiolitis: • Parent time for hospital admission and visits • Cost of travel • Lost time at work and possibly lost income and reduced job security Child discomfort: • Injections • RSV-related illnesses that are not prevented

[a] Palivizumab has been shown to reduce RSV hospitalizations by between 55% and 80%. Therefore, RSV hospitalizations will be expected in both study groups, but at a reduced rate in the palivizumab group.

Source: Data from The IMPACT RSV Study Group. (1998). Palivizumab, a humanized respiratory syncytial virus monoclonal antibody, reduces hospitalization from respiratory syncytial virus infection in high-risk infants. *Pediatrics, 102*, 531–537.

If this cost analysis were expanded to consider the costs to society, including environmental costs, the additional items to be enumerated may include items such as those in **Table 5-3**.

TABLE 5-3 Examples of Societal Costs in a Cost Analysis of Palivizumab Prophylaxis in Children Born at 32 to 35 Weeks EGA, from a Society Perspective

Prophylaxis Group	Comparison (Nonprophylaxis) Group
Lost productivity (from the perspective of the employer) of parents for time to take infants to clinic visits.	Lost productivity (from the perspective of the employer) of parents for time to spend with hospitalized child.
Lost productivity (from the perspective of the employer) of parents for time to spend with hospitalized child.	Transport to hospital:
Transport to clinic visits and hospital:	• Fuel production, transport of fuel, and pollution from use of fuel
• Fuel production, transport of fuel, and pollution from use of fuel	• Energy use of healthcare agencies
Supplies such as syringes, latex gloves, palivizumab (drug):	• Supplies and equipment used during hospitalizations (pollution-related costs)
• Pollution related to materials acquisition, manufacturing processes, distribution of supplies, packaging of supplies, and disposal	
• Energy use of healthcare agencies	
• Supplies and equipment used during hospitalizations (pollution-related costs)	

DISCUSSION QUESTIONS:

1. Consider the case of palivizumab outlined in this section. Some health leaders believe that the use of palivizumab is not the best solution to reducing RSV-related hospitalizations. Alternative approaches have been proposed, such as efforts to reduce prematurity and low birth weight, promote breastfeeding, counsel caregivers on the importance of not exposing infants to tobacco smoke, promote good hand washing, and limit infant exposure to crowds and children with respiratory infections. Select an alternative preventive approach to reducing RSV hospitalizations and outline the types of costs you would include in the

new primary prevention study arm. Be specific, and provide rationale for each cost item.

2. Select a healthcare topic of interest to you. Outline the items to include in a cost analysis when comparing a treatment-focused approach with an approach that involves primary prevention, such as promoting healthy behaviors. Describe the two approaches. Quantify the items to be included at the levels of an individual and a population. Specify the following items to be included: (a) direct and indirect healthcare costs; (b) costs to the family; and (c) costs to society, including environmental impact.

Pay for Performance

For decades fee-for-service reimbursement was the predominant approach for paying healthcare providers in the United States. Over time, with concerns of rising healthcare costs without correlative improvements in the health status of the population, the impact of paying providers on a fee-for-service basis was questioned. Studies demonstrated that fee-for-service reimbursement is often associated with higher levels of utilization, inefficiencies, and not necessarily higher quality care (Broomberg & Price, 1990; Hickson, Altemeier, & Perrin, 1987). Recognizing that the form of provider compensation often influences provider practice behaviors, third-party payers have implemented alternative compensation approaches with the intent of altering practice patterns (Quast, Sappington, & Shenkman, 2008). For example, the Social Security Amendments of 1983 changed Medicare reimbursement for inpatient services from a cost-based system to a prospective payment system (PPS) using diagnosis-related groups (DRGs) (U.S. Congress, , Office of Technology Assessment, 1985). Managed care organizations and other third-party payers have contracted with providers using per-diem, per-case, capitated, salaried, and other payment arrangements. These and other strategies have been introduced in the U.S. healthcare system to try to influence providers to contain healthcare costs and improve efficiency.

More recent provider reimbursement trends intended to influence provider practice patterns and quality of care include denial of payment to hospitals for preventable hospital errors and pay for performance (P4P) initiatives (CMS, 2007; Pear, 2007). Beginning October 1, 2008, Medicare was expected to stop paying hospitals for eight "serious preventable events," including surgical objects left in a patient, air embolism, blood incompatibility, serious bedsores, injuries from falls, urinary tract infections from catheters, vascular infections from catheters, and infection after heart-bypass graft (Consumer Reports, 2008; Pear, 2007). Some private insurance companies are following Medicare's lead and also deny payments for preventable conditions. Medicare has also designed several pay for performance initiatives targeting hospitals, physicians, and physician groups serving Medicare beneficiaries (CMS, 2007; Fenter & Lewis, 2008). The hospital quality incentive demonstration involves collecting data from hospitals on 34 measures related to five clinical conditions (CMS, 2007). These conditions include acute myocardial infarction, coronary artery bypass surgery, heart failure, community-acquired pneumonia, and hip and knee replacement (Fenter & Lewis, 2008). Hospitals that score in the top 10% for a set of quality measures receive 102% of the standard DRG payment (2% bonus) for the relevant diagnoses. Hospitals in the next 10% tier receive a 1% bonus for those diagnoses. Medicare is also exploring possible P4P programs for nursing home care, home health care, and dialysis providers (CMS, 2007).

Pay for performance programs have also been implemented in commercial health plans and Medicaid programs (Kuhmerker & Hartman, 2007; Pearson, Schneider, Kleinman, Coltin, & Singer, 2008). In Massachusetts, P4P contracts were implemented between five major payers and physician groups representing approximately 5,000 primary care physicians. Health Plan Employer Data and Information Set (HEDIS) measures served as the P4P targets (Pearson et al., 2008). Examples of HEDIS measures that were included in the initiative include breast cancer screening, cervical cancer screening, eye exams and hemoglobin A1c testing for diabetes care, and well-child visits for children and adolescents.

More than half of the state Medicaid programs had implemented pay for performance programs as of July 1, 2006 (Kuhmerker & Hartman, 2007). Approximately 70% of the Medicaid P4P programs operate within primary care case management or other managed care programs. The number of measures monitored, types of measures, and incentives used within the Medicaid programs vary from state to state. Some programs relied on only one or two measures; others focused on 10 or more measures (Kuhmerker & Hartman, 2007). The incentives used by P4P programs include payment for participation in quality improvement meetings; payment for process (payment for achievement of an activity at the individual patient level); bonuses for achievement of predetermined thresholds; tiered bonuses based on comparative ranking with other providers; bonuses for demonstration of improvement; performance-based fee schedules; differential reimbursement rates; penalties; and other approaches (Center for Health Care Strategies, 2007). State Medicaid directors believed that bonuses and differential reimbursement approaches are most effective and that penalties are the least effective approaches. Yet, penalties are the second most common approach used in state Medicaid programs. Evaluations of P4P programs need to be conducted to determine the effectiveness because few studies have been published (Pearson et al., 2008).

Pay for performance is a concept that can also be applied to personal health behaviors (Sindelar, 2008). This is of significant concern because of the substantial disease burden and healthcare and societal costs that can be attributed to health behaviors (Thorpe, Howard, & Galactionova, 2007). For example, an estimated 38% of deaths in the United States are attributable to four behaviors: smoking, poor diet, physical inactivity, and alcohol use (Woolf, 2007). The CDC estimated that 80% of diabetes, heart disease, and stroke can be prevented through reductions in obesity and smoking (Thorpe et al., 2007). Even older adults can gain significant health benefits by improving health behaviors (Goetzel et al., 2007). Older adults who engage in physical activity can reduce their risk for falls, reduce hypertension, enhance their ability to manage stress, and experience other health benefits (Goetzel et. al, 2007). Research suggests that the use of positive incentives can be effective for reducing drug use and smoking, even when using small payments (Sindelar, 2008). The cost savings to the healthcare systems and society attributable to behavior changes can far exceed the costs of financial incentives. However, it is important to consider whether incentives are fair. For example, does compensation or reward go only to those people who previously made negative health behavior decisions that they are now correcting? In addition, the issues of who funds the incentives and whether the results are lasting are also important to decisions about providing incentives to people who change health behavior patterns (Sindelar, 2008).

CASE STUDY: *Millennium Health Care*

Millennium Health Care, a hypothetical primary care case management program, entered into contractual agreements with all of its primary care providers who serve pediatric patients. The contracts specified that participating providers would be reimbursed using a fee schedule based on Current Procedural Terminology 4 (CPT-4) codes and a variation of Medicare's Resource Based Relative Value Scale (RBRVS). In addition, provider practices would be eligible to receive additional bonus payments annually under a pay for performance plan.

The measures and benchmarks established for this P4P program are listed in **Table 5-4**.

TABLE 5-4   Benchmark Measures Used in the Millennium Care P4P Program

Measure	Benchmark Value (%)	Assigned Weight (%)
1. Children with at least six well-child visits in the first 15 months of life	75	5
2. Children with at least one well-child visit in the 3rd to 6th years of life	85	5
3. Adolescents, age 12 to 19 years, with at least one well-care visit in the measurement year	60	5

(Continued)

TABLE 5-4 (*Continued*)

Measure	Benchmark Value (%)	Assigned Weight (%)
4. Children with at least one visit to the PCP between 12 and 24 months of life	97.5	5
5. Children with at least one visit to the PCP between 25 months and 6 years of age	95	5
6. Children with at least one visit to the PCP between 7 and 11 years of age	95	5
7. Preteens and teens with at least one visit to the PCP between 12 and 19 years of age	95	5
8. Child immunization rate 1: four DtaP/DT, three IPV, one MMR, three *H. influenza* type B, and three hepatitis B vaccines by the child's second birthday (subject to change as recommendations change)	80	5
9. Child immunization rate 2: same as child immunization rate 1, with the addition of one varicella (chickenpox) vaccine (VZV) and four pneumo-coccal conjugate vaccines by the second birthday	80	5
10. Adolescent immunization rate 1: percentage of children who have received the appropriate immunizations by age 13 years	70	5
11. Body mass index (BMI) computed and recorded for children 2 years of age and older	95	5
12. Healthy weight counseling performed with parents whose children are overweight or obese based on BMI	80	5
13. Children 2 years of age and older in practice are normal weight based on BMI	90	10
14. Diabetic patients documentation of blood pressure at every continuing care visit	95	5
15. Diabetic patients: HbA1c level determined twice in the past year	80	5

Measure	Benchmark Value (%)	Assigned Weight (%)
16. Diabetic patients: received annual flu vaccine	80	5
17. Asthma patients are staged	80	5
18. Asthma action plan developed when stages II–IV	80	5
19. Asthma patients received annual flu vaccine	80	5

Within this P4P system, incentives (bonuses) are distributed annually based on achievement of the predetermined thresholds for each defined measure. The maximum allowable bonus is 5% of total reimbursement for primary care services delivered to Millennium Health Care enrollees served by the respective PCPs during the year. To receive the 5% bonus, the thresholds must be achieved for all measures. If only some benchmarks are achieved, then the annual bonus would be a percentage of the 5%, based on the assigned weights in the table of measures. For example, if the provider met the benchmark levels for the first four measures in the table, then the bonus would be 20% (or one fifth) of the 5%, which is equivalent to a 1% bonus. If the practice achieved all of the thresholds except for number 13, then the provider would receive 90% of the total bonus, or a 4.5% bonus.

DISCUSSION QUESTIONS:

1. After reviewing the background information and the hypothetical case, what do you believe are the strengths of the proposed P4P plan? What are the weaknesses or limitations of this proposed P4P plan? Describe how you would propose to collect the necessary data to support this P4P initiative. What systems would be needed for documenting and monitoring these P4P measures? Describe the specifics of how the data would be captured. What types of systems, tools, or procedures would be helpful to ensure that these activities are performed by the providers? Please provide specific examples.

2. What types of problems might occur if financial rewards are given to providers for a limited number of performance achievements? For

example, if providers are rewarded for care delivery related to diabetes and asthma benchmarks only, what are the possible outcomes or unintended consequences of this approach?

3. What steps can be taken to reduce the likelihood of providers being pulled in conflicting directions by pay for performance initiatives?

4. Describe several administrative and measurement challenges related to implementing pay for performance initiatives.

5. Describe a hypothetical pay for performance initiative that would involve rewarding providers for keeping people healthy. Describe the context of the initiative, the organization or health system structure, and characteristics of the system that would be needed to help this work. Outline the reimbursement structure and proposed incentives. Identify who would receive incentives. Identify at least five sample measures and describe the process you would propose for collecting data and measuring the concepts of health.

6. How could society overcome measurement challenges when working to measure and reward population health?

7. Describe a system you would propose to create that would incentivize people to practice healthier behaviors, such as increase physical activity, stop smoking (or never start), use condoms, eat appropriate portion sizes, eat organic or pesticide-free foods, wear seat belts, and/or drive no faster than the speed limit. What mechanisms would you include to create fairness and equity and minimize fraud? How would you define at least three measures to be considered? How would you propose to have the behaviors measured? Describe the context of the program (organizational setting or system of care delivery).

References

Adams, E. K., Bronstein, J. M., & Florence, C. S. (2003). The impact of Medicaid primary care case management on office-based physician supply in Alabama and Georgia. *Inquiry, 40,* 269–282.

American Nurses Association. (2007). *ANA's principles of environmental health for nursing practice with implementation strategies.* Silver Spring, MD: Author.

American Nurses Association. (2008). Medicaid of advanced practice nursing. *Nursing World.* Retrieved from http://www.nursingworld.org/DocumentVault/GOVA/Federal/Federal-Issues/MedicaidReimbursement%20.aspx

Bengston, D. N. (1993). What is ecological economics? Retrieved from http://www.metla.fi/archive/forest/1993/09/msg00004.html

Birkmeyer, J. D., Stukel, T. A., Siewers, A. E., Goodney, P. P., Wennberg, D. E., & Lucas, F. L. (2003). Surgeon volume and operative mortality in the United States. *New England Journal of Medicine, 349*(22), 2117–2127.

Boult, C., Rassen, J., Rassen, A., Moore, R. J., & Robison, S. (2000). The effect of case management on the costs of health care for enrollees in Medicare Plus Choice plans: A randomized trial. *Journal of American Geriatric Society, 48*(8), 996–1001.

Brodsky, K. L., & Baron, R. J. (2000). A "best practices" strategy to improve quality in Medicaid managed care plans. *Journal of Urban Health, 77*(4), 592–602.

Broomberg, J., & Price, M. R. (1990). The impact of the fee-for-service reimbursement system on the utilisation of health services. *South African Medical Journal, 70,* 130–132.

Buppert, D. (2004). *Nurse practitioner's business practice and legal guide* (2nd ed.). Sudbury, MA: Jones and Bartlett Publishers.

Center for Health Care Strategies. (2007). *Physician pay-for-performance in Medicaid: A guide for states.* Retrieved from http://www.chcs.org/publications3960/publications_show.htm?doc_id=471272

Center on Budget and Policy Priorities. (2006). The number of uninsured Americans is at an all-time high. Retrieved from http://www.cbpp.org/8-29-06health.htm

Centers for Disease Control and Prevention. (2007). National Breast and Cervical Cancer Early Detection Program (NBC-CEDP): Breast and Cervical Cancer Mortality Prevention Act of 1990. Retrieved from http://www.cdc.gov/cancer/NBC-CEDP/legislation/law.htm

Centers for Disease Control and Prevention. (2008). National Breast and Cervical Cancer Early Detection Program. Retrieved from http://www.cdc.gov/cancer/NBCCEDP/

Centers for Medicare and Medicaid Services. (2005a). Breast and cervical cancer: Prevention and treatment. Retrieved from http://www.cdc.gov/cancer/nbccedp/legislation/law106–354.htm

Centers for Medicare and Medicaid Services. (2005b). Medicaid State Waiver Program Demonstration Projects-General Information-Overview. Retrieved from http://www.medicaid.gov/Medicaid-CHIP-Program-Information/By-Topics/Waivers/1115/Section-1115-Demonstrations.html/

Centers for Medicare and Medicaid Services. (2007). Details for Medicare "pay for performance" initiatives. Retrieved from http://www.cms.hhs.gov/apps/media/press/release.asp?counter=1343

Children's Hospice International. (2008). The Florida CHI PACC model. Retrieved October 7, 2008 from http://www.chionline.org/states/fl.php

City-Data.com. (2008). Hyde County, North Carolina (NC). Retrieved from http://www.city-data.com/county/Hyde_County-NC.html

Commonwealth Fund Commission on a High Performance Health System. (2008). Why not the best? Results from the national scorecard on U.S. health system performance, 2008. Retrieved from http://www.commonwealthfund.org/publications/fund-reports/2008/jul/why-not-the-best—results-from-the-national-scorecard-on-u-s—health-system-performance—2008

Community Care of North Carolina. (2008). A history of CCNC. Retrieved from http://www.communitycarenc.com/about-us/history-ccnc-rev/

Consumer Reports. (2008). Viewpoint. Hospitals will have to pay for their mistakes. Retrieved from http://www.consumerreports.org/cro/aboutus/mission/viewpoint/hospitals-will-have-to-pay-for-their-mistakes/overview/hospitals-paying-for-their-mistakes-ov.htm

Cooper, W. O., & Kuhlthau, K. (2001). Evaluating Medicaid managed care programs for children. *Ambulatory Pediatrics, 1*(2), 112–116.

Dallek, G., Parks, M., & Waxman, J. (1984). Medicaid primary care case management systems: What we've learned. *Caring, 3*(8), 23–28.

Drummond, M. F., Stoddart, G. L., & Torrance, G. L. (1989). *Methods for the economic evaluation of health care programmes.* Oxford, England: Oxford Medical Publications.

Edmarc Hospice for Children. (2008). Mission statement, vision statement, history, program and service summary, and organizational chart. Retrieved from http://www.edmarc.org/about/

Fenter, T. C., & Lewis, S.J. (2008). Pay-for-performance initiatives. *Supplement to Journal of Managed Care Pharmacy, 14*(6), S12–S16.

Ferri, R. S. (2007). Health care without harm: Nurses take action. *Medscape Today.* Retrieved from http://www.medscape.com/viewarticle/555467

Fleisher, L. (2003). Access and use of health care vary by type of Medicaid managed care program. *Changes in Health Care Financing and Organization, 6*(3), 1–3.

Goetzel, R. Z., Reynolds, K., Breslow, L., Roper, W. L., Shechter, D., Stapleton, D. C., . . . McGinnis, J. M. (2007). Health promotion in later life: It's never too late. *American Journal of Health Promotion, 21,* 1–5.

Halverson, P. K., Kaluzny, A. D., & McLaughlin, C. P. (1998). *Managed care and public health* (1st ed.). Gaithersburg, MD: Aspen.

Hickson, G. B., Altemeier, W. A., & Perrin, J. M. (1987). Physician reimbursement by salary or fee-for-service: Effect on physician practice behavior in a randomized prospective study. *Pediatrics, 80*(3), 344–350.

Highsmith, N., & Somers, S. A. (2000). Medicaid managed care. From cost savings to accountability and quality improvement. *Evaluation and the Health Professions, 23*(4), 385–396.

Holahan, J., & Suzuki, S. (2003). Medicaid managed care payment methods and capitation rates in 2001: Results of a new national survey. *Health Affairs, 22*(1), 204–218.

Hurley, R. E., & Draper, D. A. (2002). Medicaid confronts a changing managed care marketplace. *HealthCare Financing Review*, *24*(1), 11–25.

IMPACT RSV Study Group. (1998). Palivizumab, a humanized respiratory syncytial virus monoclonal antibody, reduces hospitalization from respiratory syncytial virus infection in high-risk infants. *Pediatrics*, *102*, 531–537.

Jacobson Vann, J. C. (2006). Measuring community-based case management performance: Strategies for evaluation. *Lippincott's Case Management*, *11*(3), 147–157.

Kaiser Commission on Medicaid and the Uninsured. (2001a). The basics of Medicaid, appendix 1: Medicaid legislative history, 1965–2000. Retrieved from http://kaiserfamilyfoundation.files.wordpress.com/2013/05/mrbleghistory.pdf

Kaiser Commission on Medicaid and the Uninsured. (2001b, February). Medicaid facts. Medicaid and managed care. Retrieved from http://www.kff.org/medicaid/030901-index.cfm

Kaiser Commission on Medicaid and the Uninsured. (2007a). Characteristics of the uninsured: Who is eligible for public coverage and who needs help affording coverage? Retrieved from http://www.kff.org/uninsured/7613.cfm

Kaiser Commission on Medicaid and the Uninsured. (2007b). The uninsured and their access to health care. Retrieved from http://www.kff.org/uninsured/upload/1420_09.pdf

Kaiser Commission on Medicaid and the Uninsured. (2008). Five basic facts on the uninsured. Retrieved from http://www.kff.org/uninsured/7806.cfm

Kongstvedt, P. R. (1994). *The managed health care handbook* (1st ed.). New York, NY: Aspen.

Kuhmerker, K., & Hartman, T. (2007). Pay-for-performance in state Medicaid programs: A survey of state Medicaid directors and programs. The Commonwealth Fund. Retrieved from http://www.commonwealthfund.org/publications/publications_show.htm?doc_id=472891

Landon, B. E., Huskamp, H. A., Tobias, C., & Epstein, A. M. (2000). The evolution of quality management in state Medicaid agencies: A national survey of states with comprehensive managed care programs. *Journal on Quality Improvement,* *28*(2), 72–82.

Madlin, N. (1991, March). EPO: Latest beast in the managed care menagerie. *Business and Health,* 48–53.

Mauksch, L. B., Katon, W. J., Russo, J., Tucker, S. M., Walker, E., & Cameron, J. (2003). The content of a low-income, uninsured primary care population: Including the patient agenda. *Journal of the American Board of Family Practice,* *16*(4), 278–289.

Miller, M. E., & Gengler, D. J. (1993). Medicaid care management: Kentucky's patient access and care program. *Health Care Financing Review,* *15*(1), 55–69.

Minnesota Pollution Control Agency. (1998). Arsenic in Minnesota's ground water. Retrieved from http://www.seagrant. umn.edu/newsletter/1998/03/superfund_site_still_causing_ concern.html

Moran, J. (2008). Press release: Seriously ill children's coordinated health care plan introduced. Retrieved from https://votesmart.org/public-statement/392359/seriously-ill-childrens-coordinated-health-care-plan-introduced

Muller, A., & Baker, J. A. (1996). Evaluation of the Arkansas Medicaid primary care physician management program. *Health Care Financing Review,* *17*(4), 117–133.

National Nursing Centers Consortium. (2014). http:// www.nncc.us/site/index.php/component/content/ category/12-about-nncc

Office of State Budget and Management. (2008). 2007 certified county population estimates. Retrieved from http://www. osbm.state.nc.us/ncosbm/facts_and_figures/socioeconomic_ data/population_estimates/demog/cert07pa.html

Pear, R. (2007, August 19). Medicare says it won't cover hospital errors. *New York Times* Retrieved from http:// www.nytimes.com/2007/08/19/washington/19hospital. html?_r=1&adxnnl=1&oref=slogin

Pearson, S. D., Schneider, E. C., Kleinman, K. P., Coltin, K. L., & Singer, J. A. (2008). The impact of pay-for-performance on health care quality in Massachusetts, 2001–2003. *Health Affairs,* *27*(4), 1167–1176.

Practice Greenhealth. (2008). Managing pharmaceutical waste: A 10-step blueprint for healthcare facilities in the United States. Retrieved from http://www.hercenter.org/hazmat/tenstepblueprint.pdf

Quast, T., Sappington, D. E., & Shenkman, E. (2008). Does the quality of care in Medicaid MCOs vary with the form of physician compensation? *Health Economics, 17*(4), 545–550.

Rawlings-Sekunda, J., Curtis, D., & Kaye, N. (2001). Emerging practices in Medicaid primary care case management programs. Produced for the U.S. Department of Health and Human Services, Office of the Assistant Secretary for Planning and Evaluation. Retrieved from http://aspe.hhs.gov/health/reports/pccm/index.htm

Resnick, R. (1992, September). Managed care comes to workers' compensation. *Business and Health,* 32–39.

Rowland, D., & Lyons, B. (1987). Mandatory HMO care for Milwaukee's poor. *Health Affairs, 6*(1), 87–100.

Sabatino, S. A., Coates, R. J., Uhler, R. J., Breen, N., Tangka, F., & Shaw, K. M. (2008). Disparities in mammography use among US women aged 40–64 years, by race, ethnicity, income, and health insurance status, 1993 and 2005. *Medical Care, 46*(7), 692–700.

Schneider, E. C., Landon, B. E., Tobias, C., & Epstein, A. M. (2004). Quality oversight in Medicaid primary care case management programs. *Health Affairs, 23*(6), 235–242.

Schoenman, J. A., Evans, W. N., & Schur, C. L. (1997). Primary care case management for Medicaid recipients: Evaluation of the Maryland Access to Care program. *Inquiry, 34,* 155–170.

Schulman, E. D., Sheriff, D. J., & Momany, E. T. (1997). Primary care case management and birth outcomes in the Iowa Medicaid program. *American Journal of Public Health, 87*(1), 80–84.

Shaner-McRae, H., McRae, G., & Jas, V. (2007). Environmentally safe health care agencies: Nursing's responsibility, Nightingale's legacy. *Online Journal of Issues in Nursing, 12*(2).

Sindelar, J. L. (2008). Paying for performance: The power of incentives over habits. *Health Economics, 17,* 449–451.

Smith, W. R., Cotter, J. J., McClish, D. K., Bovbjerg, V. E., & Rossiter, L. F. (2000). Access, satisfaction, and utilization in two forms of Medicaid managed care. *Clinical Performance and Quality Health Care, 8*(3), 150–157.

Smith, W. R., Cotter, J. J., & Rossiter, L. F. (1996). System change: Quality assessment and improvement for Medicaid managed care. *Health Care Financing Review, 17*(4), 97–115.

Sofaer, S, Woolley, S. F., Kenney, K. A., Kreling, B., & Mauery, D. R. (1998). Meeting the challenge of serving people with disabilities: A resource guide for assessing the performance of managed care organizations. Center for Health Outcomes Improvement Research, Center for Health Policy Research. Retrieved from http://www.aspe.hhs.gov/daltcp/reports/resource.htm

Social Security Act, Pub. L. 74-271, 49 Stat. 620. Enacted August 14, 1935.

Tainter, J. A. (1996). Complexity, problem solving, and sustainable societies. In *Getting down to earth: Practical applications of ecological economics*. Retrieved from http://www.dieoff.org/page134.htm

Thorpe, K. E., Howard, D. H., & Galactionova, K. (2007). Differences in disease prevalence as a source of the U.S.-European health care spending gap. *Health Affairs, Web Exclusive*, w678–w686.

Torrisi, D. L., & Hansen-Turton, T. (2005). *Community and nurse-managed health centers: Getting them started and keeping them going. A National Nursing Centers Consortium Guide.* New York, NY: Springer.

Tufts Managed Care Institute. (1998). Managed care models and products. Retrieved from http://free.influence2.org/m/managed-care-models-and-products-tufts-health-care-institute-home–w1007/

Ury, W., & Fisher, R. (1988). *Getting to yes: Negotiating agreement without giving in.* The Harvard Negotiating Project. New York, NY: Penguin.

U.S. Census Bureau. (2007). Income, poverty, and health insurance coverage in the United States: 2006. U.S. Department of Commerce, Economics and Statistics Administration. Retrieved from http://www.census.gov/prod/2007pubs/p60–233.pdf

U.S. Congress, Office of Technology Assessment. (1985, October). *Medicare's prospective payment system: Strategies for evaluating cost, quality, and medical technology* (OTA-H-262). Washington, DC: U.S. Government Printing Office. Retrieved from http://govinfo.library.unt.edu/ota/Ota_4/DATA/1985/8516.PDF

U.S. Department of Health and Human Services. (2008). The 2008 HHS poverty guidelines. Retrieved from http://aspe.hhs.gov/poverty/08Poverty.shtml

U.S. Department of Health and Human Services, Office of Inspector General. (2005). Status of the rural health clinic program. Retrieved from http://oig.hhs.gov/oei/reports/oei-05-03-00170.pdf

Vanhook, P. M. (2007). Cost-utility analysis: A method of quantifying the value of registered nurses. *Online Journal of Issues in Nursing, 12*(3). Retrieved from http://www.nursingworld.org/MainMenuCategories/ANAMarketplace/ANAPeriodicals/OJIN/TableofContents/Volume122007/No3Sept07/CostUtilityAnalysis.aspx

Wegner, S., Jacobson Vann, J., Liu, G., Byrns, P., Cypra, C., Campbell, W., & Stiles, A. (2004). Direct cost analysis of palivizumab treatment in a cohort of at-risk children: Evidence from the North Carolina Medicaid program. *Pediatrics, 114*(6), 1612–1619.

White, C. (2007). Health care spending growth: How different is the United States from the rest of the OECD? *Health Affairs, 26*(1), 154–161.

Williams, S. J., & Torrens, P.R. (1993). *Introduction to health services* (4th ed.). Albany, NY: Delmar.

Williams, S. J., & Torrens, P. R. (2002). *Introduction to health services* (5th ed.). Albany, NY: Delmar.

Williamson, E. (2006, February 16). Study links 700 deaths yearly to Md. plants. *Washington Post.* Retrieved from http://www.washingtonpost.com/wp-dyn/content/article/2006/02/15/AR2006021502582_pf.html

Wilper, A. P, Woolhandler, S., Lasser, K. E., McCormick, D., Bor, D. H., & Himmelstein, D. U. (2008). A national study of chronic disease prevalence and access to care in uninsured U.S. adults. *Annals of Internal Medicine, 149*(3), 170–176.

Wisconsin Department of Health Services. (2008). Wisconsin Medicaid, managed care. Retrieved from http://www.dhs.wisconsin.gov/bdds/waivermanual/Archive/waiverch07_08.pdf

Woolf, S. H. (2007). Potential health and economic consequences of misplaced priorities. *Journal of American Medical Association, 297*(5), 523–526.

Zuckerman, S., Brennan, N., & Yemane, A. (2002). Has Medicaid managed care affected beneficiary access and use? *Inquiry, 39*(3), 221–242.

CHAPTER 6

Quality Management

Linda Searle Leach, PhD, RN, NEA-BC, CNL

Learning Objectives

1. Discuss the importance of quality management and the principles of quality improvement to the role of advanced practice nurses in transforming healthcare systems.
2. Conduct a root cause analysis that identifies the multiple causal factors that contribute to the outcome or challenge posed by a healthcare case study.
3. Design a plan, do, study, act (PDSA) cycle for the specified area identified for improvement.
4. Explain the role of peer review in monitoring quality and performance standards.

The Healthcare Chasm

"Between the health care we have and the care we could have lies not just a gap but a chasm" (Institute of Medicine [IOM], 2001, p. 1). The word *chasm* implies a notable divide between what U.S. health care is and what it should be. *Crossing the Quality*

Chasm: A New Health System for the 21st Century is the second in a series of reports produced by the Institute of Medicine (IOM) about health care in the United States (IOM, 2001). *Crossing the Quality Chasm*, a guide to achieving high-quality care through redesigning the healthcare delivery system, addresses the needed improvements. Noteworthy in the report is the perspective that to reduce the burden of illness, injury, and disability in the United States, professionals from all disciplines, including direct care providers, administrators, and educators—indeed, involvement from the system as a whole—are required to participate.

The impetus for detailing the quality issues emerged in the aftermath of public awareness of the extent and serious nature of medical errors throughout the United States. With patient safety as a galvanizing focus of reform, the quality chasm report featured the gaps in care delivery and identified the following quality problems:

- Forty-one million uninsured Americans exhibit consistently worse clinical outcomes than the insured do and are at increased risk of dying prematurely.
- Eighteen thousand Americans die each year from heart attacks because they did not receive preventive medication.
- More than 50% of patients with diabetes, hypertension, tobacco addiction, hyperlipidemia, congestive heart failure, asthma, depression, and/or chronic atrial fibrillation are managed inadequately.
- Patients are being harmed; care needs are not being met.
- Care is not consistently based on scientific evidence.
- New technologies are not appropriately and safely used.
- Patient information is fragmented among providers.
- Costs continue to escalate.
- Healthcare remains inaccessible to an extensive number of Americans who are underinsured or without health insurance (IOM, 2001).

The report identifies three types of quality problems: overuse, misuse, and underuse. Overuse of healthcare technologies such as medications or frequent use of treatments when their use is questionable or there is no evidence of benefit represents one type of problem with the quality of care. Examples of overuse include prescribing antibiotics for viral bronchitis and performing excessive or inappropriate surgeries. The problem of misuse involves using technologies incorrectly, for example, combining medications inadvertently to create a preventable adverse drug event. In contrast, the underuse of available and beneficial healthcare procedures, medications, or treatments is exemplified by lack of screening for breast cancer with mammograms and vaccinations not given.

Although the increase in quality improvement activities and the focus on the quality of health over the last decade are unparalleled in the history of the U.S. healthcare system, the public's perception of the healthcare system as trustworthy and honest is trending downward. A Harris poll reported that 35% of adults viewed hospitals as trustworthy and honest in 2004, 34% in 2005, and the percentage declined further to 29% in 2010 (Harris Interactive, 2010). Medical errors continue to occur and affect 1.5 million people each year. Two million people are affected by hospital-acquired infections, which contribute to 90,000 deaths (IOM, 2007; Joint Commission, 2003). Most recently, in a poll sponsored by the Robert Wood Johnson Foundation, approximately half of Americans rated the quality of health care in the United States as low, a C or D on a report card scale, and 11% gave it a failing (F) grade (Blendon, 2011). One of the resounding concerns about the gap in quality was a 17-year lag between discovery of new technologies and more effective treatments and their implementation in routine patient care. To improve how the system is organized and reduce costs and variation in health outcomes, major reform rather than incremental change is needed.

A new healthcare system for the 21st century was envisioned as safe, effective, patient-centered, timely, equitable, and efficient (IOM, 2001). These six aims provide the contemporary view of the dimensions of quality health care and serve as the framework for transformational change. The IOM report emphasizes the importance of the commitment to a shared vision of health care that fulfills these six aims by all who have a stake in health care.

Quality Defined

Quality is considered to be a complex concept, and those involved in health care, including providers, patients, and payers, may define it differently. The IOM (1999) definition of quality is "the degree to which health services for individuals and populations increase the likelihood of desired health outcomes and are consistent with current professional knowledge" (p. 4). A widely known conceptualization of quality based on the work of Donabedian (1980) includes structure, process, and outcome elements. Measuring quality in relation to structure includes examining the characteristics of individuals providing care, care delivery settings, equipment, organization, and adequacy of resources such as staffing. Processes of care are the actions that encompass the delivery of care and are delineated as appropriateness (the right care) and skill (carried out well). Outcomes from care are measures of goal achievement such as health status and include costs of care and patient satisfaction. Outcomes must be linked to the care process or attributed to the care provided to indicate care quality. Outcomes of health status such as pain relief and functional status are influenced by factors beyond care delivery, such as environmental influences and genetic makeup; these influencing factors reflect individual uniqueness that can contribute to variation in healthcare outcomes.

Improving the quality of care was the main objective of the quality chasm report, and patient safety is featured as a key component of quality (IOM, 2001). The essential improvements in the quality of healthcare delivery in the United States that were identified include the following:

- Care that is responsive to patients' needs and preferences
- Care that is patient-centered with patients' participating in decision making
- Care that is based on evidence
- Standardized practice based on scientific and best evidence to reduce variability

Patient needs and preferences is an evolving area that has been assisted by the extent of information available on the Internet.

Ready access to a wealth of information informs patients of their alternatives and choices. The foundation of what is known about patient preferences comes from the landmark study describing what patients really want (Gerteis, Edgman-Levetan, & Daley, 1993). In this study, patients described quality care as follows:

- Care that is technical, therapeutic, appropriate, and efficient and that can be assessed by professional standards, clinical outcomes, and technical measures
- Care that is respectful of patients' values, preferences, and expressed needs
- Care that is coordinated and services that are integrated within a healthcare setting: communication is coordinated between patient and providers; information is shared and is accurate, timely, and appropriate; education about long-term implications is provided; coordination includes transition and continuity from one location/episode of care to another
- Physical care, comfort, and the alleviation of pain
- Emotional support and alleviation of fears and anxiety
- Involvement of family and friends
- Quality of the patient's experience that can be assessed only by patients themselves

Quality Management

As mentioned earlier, despite the increase in quality improvement activities and a focus on the quality of health, the public's perception of the health system continues to decline. To achieve the vision of a redesigned healthcare system, new and better ways to care for patients are needed. Quality management is an improvement process, a way of systematically evaluating and continuously improving products and services to achieve better performance (Spath, 2009). Quality management in health care has been influenced by the continuous improvement approaches and statistical quality control processes used in business and manufacturing (Spath, 2009).

Principles of Quality Improvement

The basic activities of managing quality improvement (QI) focus on measurement, assessment, and improvement activities. Measurement provides data about the quality of patient care. These results are compared to a standard or performance expectation. The level of performance shows the performance gap if one exists and guides the improvement approach. Improvement processes are based on key principles:

- Quality should be defined by the consumer of health care.
- Variation in the process of care must be understood and reduced.
- Top management must be committed to improvement.
- Change and improvement must be continuous and part of care delivery.
- Training and education of all employees must be ongoing.
- Change and growth through collaboration, cooperation, and compromise are fostered.

THE MODEL FOR IMPROVEMENT

A framework that is being used to accelerate improvement in many healthcare organizations is the Model for Improvement (Langley, Nolan, Nolan, Norman, & Provost, 2009). Models guide individuals and groups and facilitate their abilities to engage in QI. The Model for Improvement has two components. The first consists of asking three strategic questions that make explicit the aim of the QI work, delineate the way to measure change, and identify change that will be an improvement (Langley et al., 2009). The second component is the process of testing, implementing, and spreading the change using the Plan-Do-Study-Act (PDSA) cycle (Deming, 1986).

The Model for Improvement starts with these three questions, which can be addressed in any order:

1. What are we trying to accomplish?
2. How will we know that a change is an improvement?
3. What change can we make that will result in improvement?

Once there is a plan for change, the PDSA cycle of action learning is used to guide the improvement process. The cycle involves trying the change, observing the results, and acting on what is learned from testing the change. The PDSA approach is intended to be a rapid cycle so that ideas are tested for a brief period and evaluated for their usefulness. In a small way or in a localized area, the idea is piloted. Then the test, with the results and learning of taking action, is shared for wider use. Efficiency is inherent in this approach. The PDSA cycle is detailed in **Figure 6-1**.

ROOT CAUSE ANALYSIS

Another method for quality improvement is root cause analysis (RCA). An RCA is a problem-solving method directed at finding the underlying and direct causes of problems or adverse events. An RCA is a tool to elicit all the possible causes contributing to an effect or problem. RCAs are also called cause-and-effect diagrams, Ishikawa diagrams, and fishbone diagrams because the lines between the cause categories resemble the backbone of a fish (see **Figure 6-2**).

This widely used tool was developed in the 1940s by Karu Ishikawa to identify sources of process variation (Ishikawa, 1987). The first step in conducting an RCA using a fishbone diagram is to determine the effect or problem. An *effect* can be a positive circumstance, whereas *problem* denotes a negative situation. The RCA process facilitates identifying the major factors that contribute to the problem using the categories of environment, procedures, equipment, and people as major factors. More categories may be added for complex problems. Each category is a factor from which subfactors that influence this cause of the problem are identified. These are added to the arm connected to the major category until all possible contributing causes are listed. This process is repeated for each major factor. When those working on the diagram have diverse experiences and perspectives of the problem, the diagram can reflect a fuller and more comprehensive view of the varied contributors that further clarifies the scope of the problem.

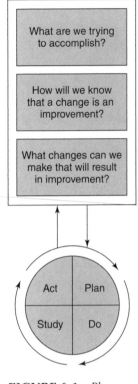

FIGURE 6-1 Plan-Do-Study-Act rapid cycle change process of quality improvement.
Source: Modified from Langley, G. L., Nolan, K. M., Nolan, T. W., Norman, C. L., & Provost, L. P. (2009). *The improvement guide: A practical approach to enhancing organizational performance* (2nd ed.). San Francisco, CA: Jossey-Bass Publishers.

Plan: Selecting Changes

All improvement requires making changes, but not all changes result in improvement. Organizations therefore must identify the changes that are most likely to result in improvement.

SETTING AIMS

Improvement requires setting aims. The aim should be time-specific and measurable; it should also define the specific population of patients that will be affected.

ESTABLISHING MEASURES

Teams use quantitative measures to determine whether a specific change actually leads to an improvement.

Do: Conducting the Test/Implementing a Change

The Plan-Do-Study-Act (PDSA) cycle is shorthand for testing a change in the real work setting—by planning it, trying it, observing the results, and acting on what is learned. This is the scientific method used for action-oriented learning.

Study: Analyzing, Comparing, Learning from Testing Changes

After testing a change on a small scale, learning from each test, and refining the change through several PDSA cycles, the team can implement the change on a broader scale—for example, for an entire pilot population or on an entire unit.

Act: Spreading Changes

Identify any modifications needed. After successful implementation of a change or package of changes for a pilot population or an entire unit, the team can spread the changes to other parts of the organization or in other organizations.

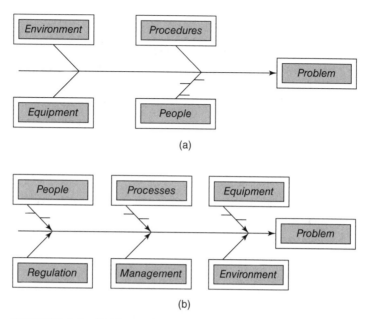

FIGURE 6-2 Fishbone diagram for root cause analysis.

Prior to pursuing solutions to the underlying causes identified in an RCA, the Five Whys should be employed. The Five Whys is a tool that enables exploration of contributing factors by digging deeper and asking why successively, starting with the problem. For example, if the problem identified is "The alarm on a patient's EKG telemetry monitor was turned off," then the first why question would be, "Why was the alarm turned off?" The answer might be because the alarm was sounding all the time. The second why question would be, "Why was the alarm sounding off all the time?" If the answer is because the patient was restless, then the third why question would be, "Why was the patient restless?" If the answer is because the patient was symptomatic and becoming hypoxic, then the fourth why question would be, "Why was the patient becoming hypoxic?" The answer might be because no action was taken when the patient's heart rate increased and oxygen saturation decreased slightly. The fifth why question would be, "Why was no action taken?" This process is designed to elucidate pertinent contributing factors that may not be readily identified.

EXTERNAL DRIVERS OF HEALTHCARE QUALITY

Healthcare quality management is influenced by external forces. External drivers of quality are government regulations, accreditation groups, and purchasers of healthcare services. Almost all healthcare organizations operate under quality directives that require improvement activities to achieve certification or to adhere to legislative regulations.

Regulations

Regulations include both federal and state programs and rules; most regulations are state level, and they differ from state to state. However, healthcare organizations that receive money from the federal government for health services provided must adhere to federal and state regulations. The Centers for Medicare and Medicaid Services (CMS) is one source of federal regulations. The change to reduced reimbursement for readmissions within 30 days among chronic cardiac patients is one example of a regulation designed to drive quality.

Accreditation

Another key force influencing healthcare quality is accreditation and the performance standards required to earn it. The function of accrediting bodies and the role of accreditation of a healthcare organization is to improve care. The Joint Commission is the most well known accrediting body for healthcare organizations. It accredits hospitals, home health agencies, ambulatory care facilities, long-term care centers, behavioral health services, and more. The accreditation standards include requirements for quality measurement, assessment, and improvement activities. Accreditation is voluntary, although the number of purchasers and government bodies requiring it is growing (Spath, 2009). (See **Table 6-1**.)

The Joint Commission propagated the need for systematic QI efforts that emphasize evaluating the results of improvement initiatives. It also developed performance measures (ORYX) for clinical outcomes of selected measures. Subsequently, the Joint Commission designed and tested a set of hospital core measures

TABLE 6-1 Accreditation Programs in Health Care

Accreditation Group	Website	Organizations and Programs Accredited
Accreditation Association for Ambulatory Health Care	http://www.aaahc.org	Hospital-affiliated ambulatory care facilities and freestanding facilities, including university student health centers
Accreditation Commission for Health Care	http://www.achc.org	Home healthcare providers, including durable medical equipment companies
American Accreditation HealthCare Commission	http://www.urac.org	Health plans, credentials verification organizations, independent review organizations, and others; also accredits specific functions in healthcare organizations such as case management, disease management
American Association for Accreditation of Ambulatory Surgery Facilities	http://www.aaaasf.org	Ambulatory surgery facilities
American Association of Blood Banks (AABB)	http://www.aabb.org	Freestanding and provider-based blood banks, transfusion services, and blood donation centers
College of American Pathologists	http://www.cap.org	Laboratory Accreditation Program Biorepository Accreditation Program Reproductive Accreditation Program Forensic Drug Testing Accreditation Program
Commission on Accreditation of Rehabilitation Facilities	http://www.carf.org	Freestanding and provider-based medical rehabilitation and human service programs, such as behavioral health, child and youth services, and opioid treatment

(Continued)

TABLE 6-1 Accreditation Programs in Health Care (*Continued*)

Accreditation Group	Website	Organizations and Programs Accredited
Commission on Cancer of the American College of Surgeons	http://www.facs. org/cancer/coc/ approval.html	Cancer programs at hospitals and freestanding treatment centers
Community Health Accreditation Program	http://www. chapinc.org	Community-based health services, including home health agencies, hospices, and home medical equipment providers
Accreditation Commission for Health Care	http://www.achc. org/programs/ dmepos	Providers of durable medical equipment, prosthetics, and supplies (e.g. diabetic, ostomy, incontinence) such as pharmacies, home care agencies, podiatrists, and orthopaedic surgeons
Continuing Care Accreditation Commission	http://www.carf. org/Accreditation/	Continuing care retirement communities and aging services networks that are part of home, community, or hospital-based systems
Diagnostic Modality Accreditation Program of the American College of Radiology	http://www.acr.org http://www.acr. org/~/media/ ACR/Documents/ Accreditation/ Apply/ DiagnosticReqs.pdf	Freestanding and provider-based imaging services, including radiology and nuclear medicine
DNV Healthcare	http://www.dnv. com/industry/ healthcare	Hospitals
Healthcare Facilities Accreditation Program of the American Osteopathic Association	http://www.hfap. org	Hospitals, hospital-based laboratories, ambulatory care/surgery, mental health, substance, abuse, and physical rehabilitation medicine facilities
Healthcare Quality Association on Accreditation	http://www.hqaa. org	Durable medical equipment providers

Accreditation Group	Website	Organizations and Programs Accredited
Intersocietal Accreditation Commission	http://www.intersocietal.org/intersocietal.htm	Freestanding and provider-based nuclear medicine and nuclear cardiology laboratories
Joint Commission	http://www.jointcommission.org	General, psychiatric, children's, and rehabilitation hospitals; critical access hospitals; medical equipment services, hospice services, and other home care organizations; nursing homes and long-term care facilities; behavioral health organizations, addiction services; rehabilitation centers, group practices, office-based surgeries, and other ambulatory care providers; and independent or freestanding laboratories
National Commission on Correctional Health Care	http://www.ncchc.org	Healthcare services in jails, prisons, and juvenile confinement facilities
National Committee for Quality Assurance	http://www.ncqa.org	Managed care and preferred provider organizations, managed behavioral healthcare organizations, and disease management programs

Source: Reprinted by permission of Health Administration Press. Spath, P. (2009). *Introduction to healthcare quality management.* Chicago, IL: Health Administration Press.

for major diagnoses, including acute myocardial infarction, heart failure, community-acquired pneumonia, pregnancy, and surgical infection prevention.

The Joint Commission requires each patient has a comprehensive patient safety plan. Mechanisms for reporting, analyzing, and preventing medical errors form the framework. Serious adverse events (formerly referred to as sentinel events), unexpected occurrences involving death or serious injury or the risk thereof, are a featured component of the patient safety plan (Joint Commission, 2003).

In 2003, the Joint Commission established a national Nursing Advisory Committee. Nurses who serve on the committee advise about safety and quality care issues. The Joint Commission includes nurse-sensitive measures in the accreditation process for hospitals. Through a voluntary consensus process, the National Quality Forum adopted 15 national standards about nurse-sensitive care that have been endorsed by the Joint Commission. Advanced practice nurses (APNs) need to remain current with changes in the standards used to evaluate the quality of care. Being knowledgeable about safety standards and the documentation required in delivering care is part of APNs' role in leading change and improving quality.

Purchasers

Healthcare quality is influenced by purchasers of healthcare services. The largest purchaser is the federal government. Healthcare organizations that participate in government programs such as Medicare must meet quality requirements that include reporting on the quality of care provided. Requirements for provider categories, such as eligibility for particular activities, are included in the federal regulation Conditions of Participation. These conditions form a contract between the government and the purchaser of healthcare services.

Private insurers are also purchasers of health care in the United States. They tend to use government regulations and accreditation standards for their quality management requirements. Their requirements are explicated in provider contracts and specify the provider's responsibility for quality management.

Approaches to Monitor and Improve Healthcare Quality

STANDARDS OF CARE

Standards of care are one way to describe the expected and acceptable actions in health care. Standards can be used to both monitor and improve quality. A standard is an authoritative statement of acceptable actions by healthcare organizations and individual healthcare providers. The authority of the statement emerges from the expert authority of professional associations, the legal authority of state and federal laws, including nurse practice acts, and regulations enacted by healthcare organizations, accrediting bodies, and state and federal agencies. Standards should reflect scientific knowledge and be based on evidence. Some standards of care describe practice, such as nursing practice, and convey how care is delivered and the scope of practice, delineating what nursing functions are appropriate. Standards of professional performance convey the appropriate actions for a role such as ethical conduct.

POLICIES AND PROCEDURES

Policies and procedures are local decisions made within a healthcare organization to specify rules and the way care should be delivered. They should be developed based on evidence and should incorporate scientific knowledge. Policies and procedures contribute to quality by providing consistency in the specified approaches to care and a means to evaluate the extent to which they are followed.

LICENSURE AND CREDENTIALING

Verification of the licensure of nurses, physicians, and allied health workers is a key component of ensuring quality in healthcare organizations. Licensure is dictated by state law. Being awarded a license to practice indicates an individual has met the minimum standards set by the state's practice act to ensure the public's safety. A healthcare organization is responsible for verifying that individuals have current licenses, or the organization can be considered complicit in breaking the law by allowing persons to practice without a license.

Credentialing is a more comprehensive verification and judgment through review of specified criteria. Credentialing is a method of monitoring the expected and appropriate preparation of healthcare providers who want to be awarded privileges to practice in the organization, to admit patients, or to be eligible for participating in Medicare or Medicaid. The credentialing process involves review of licensure, hospital privileges, Drug Enforcement Administration registration, education and board certification, malpractice insurance, liability claims history, national practitioner Data Bank queries, medical board sanctions, Medicare and/or Medicaid sanctions, and provider applications. Practitioners are required to contribute to the process of credentials review and to establish the criteria for approving provider credentials.

UTILIZATION REVIEW AND MANAGEMENT

Healthcare organizations use utilization review and management to evaluate the necessity, appropriateness, and efficiency of healthcare services for individual patients and patient populations. Utilization data, drawn mostly from medical records, inform administration about use of services as well as outcomes and the volume of services in relation to budgets and reimbursement. Utilization review is used to assess the necessity and extent of services and to evaluate data in relation to patient outcomes. Utilization review also contributes data for financial analysis relative to budgeted services, procedures, and reimbursement.

PEER REVIEW

Healthcare professionals evaluate members of their discipline in a process called clinical peer review. Peer review helps improve the quality and safety of care by ensuring physician competency and that care given is within medicine's scope of practice. It also contributes to decreasing liability associated with malpractice and meeting regulatory requirements that in the United States include accreditation, licensure, and Medicare participation. Peer review also supports the other processes that healthcare organizations have in place to ensure that physicians are competent and practice within the boundaries of professionally accepted norms.

When APNs are credentialed to provide care according to their nursing scope of practice, they begin the peer review process. Healthcare organizations use a process to review licensure and requirements of APNs' advanced practice scope. Organizations are interested in neutralizing any vulnerability to malpractice actions and ensuring that a practitioner complies with regulations prior to being granted privileges to practice. Peer review among nurses is not fully established as a mechanism to ensure competency. Most APNs are employed at the organization where they practice, and evaluation is performance-based according to the professional job description. Physicians typically operate outside those employment ties and thus a mechanism for performance evaluation through peer review is used.

One implication for APNs is for them to participate in peer review of physician partners. As team-based care becomes a standard for delivery, not only will individuals need to receive performance feedback from others in their discipline but also from the team. When the team is interprofessional, then representative members of the team should participate in team reviews.

RISK MANAGEMENT

Quality improvement activities can be related to risk management interventions and risk reduction processes. QI activities should minimize liability of providers and institutions when they improve the quality of care, reduce errors, and avoid adverse outcomes (IOM, 2001). The goal of risk management is a healthcare environment that is both safe and effective in which losses to the organization are prevented or reduced (Youngberg & Weber, 1997). Errors and incidents are evaluated relative to risk. Risk managers intervene when patients incur injuries or harm. Effective risk management can reduce risk of patient injury and contribute to patient safety improvements. The focus is to minimize the financial losses related to malpractice and legal actions.

National Committee for Quality Assurance

The National Committee for Quality Assurance (NCQA) began developing accreditation programs and performance measures for managed care organizations in 1990. NCQA was responsible for holding health maintenance organizations (HMOs) accountable for the quality of the services provided. This led to a group of performance measures for HMOs called the Health Plan Employer Data and Information Set (HEDIS). Through the NCQA, a database for HEDIS measures called the Quality

Compass was established and has subsequently become the Health Plan Report Card on the NCQA website.

HEDIS measures define the data needed for analysis of more than 50 areas of health plan performance. The measures are designed to evaluate six categories: access and availability, effectiveness of care, utilization of services, member satisfaction, cost of care, and health plan stability. HEDIS measures contribute about 25% of a health plan's score for performance. HEDIS measures are the framework for data used to evaluate care provided by a health plan. APNs need to understand these measures and how their practice might influence a plan's performance.

NCQA accredits managed care organizations, managed behavioral health organizations, physician organizations, credentials verification organizations, preferred provider organizations, new health plans, the Veterans Administration Human Research Protection Accreditation Program, and the Partnership for Human Research Protections Accreditation Program. Accreditors review program structure, operations, relationships, effects on providers and members, performance measurement, and delegation in each of the following areas: quality management and improvement, utilization management, credentialing and recredentialing, member rights and responsibilities, preventive health services, and medical records. More than 50% of managed care plans in the United States go through this certification process, and current listings of accredited entities are provided on the NCQA website. APNs are likely to contribute to accreditation where they are employed in delivering care and measuring performance according to established criteria.

Institute for Healthcare Improvement

The Institute for Healthcare Improvement (IHI) began in 1991 as a safety initiative as a reaction to the IOM's efforts to focus attention on patient safety. The mission of IHI is to provide the energy, knowledge, and support for an ongoing campaign to improve health care throughout the world (Finkelman & Kenner, 2010). The approach IHI uses is to develop and implement innovations likely to influence preventable deaths and other adverse events. A campaign approach to involve hospitals in "saving 100,000 lives" brought extensive voluntary involvement, including enrollment of 3,000 hospitals in the United States. Rapid response teams and a bundle of interventions to prevent ventilator-associated pneumonia were two of the initial safety initiatives. Additional interventions were included in the subsequent 5 Million Lives campaign.

IHI continues to be a resource for informing about complex problems, measuring results from improvement changes, and sharing global experiences to advance improvement efforts. The institute also provides online educational opportunities to develop knowledge and new skills related to safety and improvement science. IHI is a central network for sharing knowledge about quality improvement. APNs can benefit from the reports of quality efforts contributed on a variety of topics and from diverse healthcare settings. APNs can lead quality improvement projects and use the wide array of resources that IHI provides to facilitate measurement, data collection, analysis, and dissemination. IHI offers a number of classes online that APNs can use to expand their knowledge or coordinate learning for colleagues and project team members. Participating and presenting at the annual IHI conference on quality is another way for APNs to lead change through quality improvement.

Leading Change, Advancing Health: The IOM *Future of Nursing* Report

The IOM's report, *Future of Nursing: Leading Change, Advancing Health*, is one of the most widely viewed online, accessible reports in the history of the IOM (Hassmiller, 2012). As a result of the Affordable Care Act (ACA), increased emphasis is placed on preparing for the provision of health care to millions more Americans. In this context, the IOM report is a clarion call to envision the role of nurses, the role of nursing education, and preparation of nurses in ways that will maximize their contribution and effectiveness. The future of nursing will evolve from an unwavering advocacy for quality patient care, safe passage for patients and families in every healthcare episode, and improved outcomes that are less costly and consistent with patient expectations. The implications for advanced practice nurses are: (1) emphasis on how well prepared nurses are and how their abilities to deliver care are foundational to healthcare quality, and (2) opportunities to assume key roles as leaders and team members in establishing a patient-centric healthcare system. In particular, the recommendation to expand opportunities for nurses to lead and diffuse collaborative improvement efforts indicates the importance of nurses knowing quality improvement principles and how to manage quality processes to improve health outcomes and reduce costs.

APNs are essential to the transformation of the healthcare system. They collaborate with patients and families as partners in care. APNs need to be able to use new knowledge to analyze outcomes of nursing interventions, evaluate team-based care delivery, and initiate change (American Association of Colleges of Nursing, 2011). The National Research Council's report, *Health Professions Education: A Bridge to Quality* (2003), identified five core competencies that should be a part of the educational preparation for health professionals: (1) apply QI and make it effective; (2) identify errors and hazards in care; (3) understand and implement basic safety design principles, such as standardization and simplification; (4) understand and measure quality of care in terms of structure, process, and outcomes; and (5) design and test interventions to change processes and systems of care, with the objective of improving quality. These educational standards can be a guide for practicing nurses as they identify learning needs and plan for their professional development.

National Healthcare Quality and Disparities Reports

Another approach to learning and keeping up-to-date with progress in quality improvements and areas of concern is through the National Healthcare Quality and Disparities Reports. These are produced by and are available from the Agency for Healthcare Research and Quality (AHRQ) at http://www.ahrq.gov. Reports are prepared annually and address the following: the status of healthcare quality and disparities in the United States, how healthcare quality and disparities have changed over time, and where the need to improve healthcare quality and reduce disparities is greatest. The most recent report presents the national priorities for quality improvement in health care, analysis of care received by older Americans, and the areas targeted for more progress.

CASE STUDY: *The Josie King Story, 2002*

Josie King did not survive her hospital stay. She died from dehydration and administration of a contraindicated narcotic that resulted in cardiac arrest and brain death. She was 18 months old. Her death and the errors involved were preventable. For parents, the loss of their child is a tragedy. Coping with the realization that such a loss was preventable seems insurmountable. Perhaps even worse was knowing that something was seriously wrong before the child succumbed, as happened to Sorrel King, Josie's mother. This is her story too.

Josie was admitted to pediatric intensive care at Johns Hopkins Medical Center in Baltimore, Maryland, for second- and third-degree burns she incurred when she climbed into a bath that was heated too hot by a faulty water heater in the Kings' home. During the 10 days that Josie was in the PICU, she received attentive care that was family-centered and inclusive of Sorrel, who was with her every minute. Josie recovered quickly as the burns healed well. Her discharge seemed imminent after being transferred to an intermediate care unit.

Josie's clinical decline became apparent to Sorrel when the toddler became desperately thirsty, sucking intensely on a washcloth during her bath and screaming out for a drink when she saw one. Then, Sorrel saw that Josie's eyes rolled back in her head when she put her to bed. Sorrel asked the nurse to call the doctor but received reassurance that this was not uncommon and that Josie's vital signs were stable. Sorrel asked another nurse to look at Josie because Josie had never done this before. She was reassured again that Josie was fine and that it would be okay for Sorrel to go home to sleep that night.

Sorrel called two times during the night and returned early the next morning. After one look at Josie, she demanded that a physician come immediately. Two shots of Narcan (naloxone) were given along with verbal orders for there to be no narcotics administered. Josie was allowed to have fluids and consumed nearly a half liter of juice. Later than morning, a nurse who Sorrel thought had been acting odd, gave Josie an injection of methadone, and in response to Sorrel's objection, the nurse said the orders for Josie had been changed.

Josie's heart stopped and her eyes fixed. She did not regain consciousness and was removed from life support 2 days later after her two brothers and sister were able to see her and say good-bye.

When complex healthcare organizations are viewed as systems, the strategy of minimizing the risk of harm to patients through improving the safety of the system of care delivery and ensuring system effectiveness becomes paramount. Most healthcare errors are systemic and not caused by the poor performance of clinicians (Schyve, 2005). Relying on individual providers and perfect performance to keep patients safe is not adequate in highly complex systems that involve interdependent system components. Acknowledging that human factors influence human behavior is fundamental to designing safe care delivery systems. Human factors are a condition of being human. Examples of human factors include fatigue, cognitive overload, inability to focus on multiple pieces of information, and distraction. Organizational cultures of safety are characterized by safe systems that minimize human fallibilities. They are designed to protect against human errors. Organizations that create cultures of safety foster a learning environment and promote healthy work environments.

Communication failures are the most frequently reported reasons for sentinel events, unexpected occurrences that involve death or serious injury, now more commonly called serious adverse events. They were called *sentinel* because they signal that immediate investigation or response is needed (Joint Commission, 2003). In the case of Josie King, the hospital took several actions that were unusual and atypical in circumstances involving sentinel events. First, it approached the family and apologized for the death of the Kings' daughter. Most hospitals and clinicians have in the past avoided encounters that might convey culpability, sometimes avoiding any contact with the parties involved or relying on legal representatives for resolution. Second, the hospital conveyed its commitment to determine what had gone wrong and then to fully disclose what it found. Third, it established the Josie King Patient Safety Foundation to support activities that advance patient safety and involve the public and professionals in learning about error prevention. Fourth, it created a new role, patient safety officer, to lead the efforts to learn.

The Institute for Healthcare Improvement invited Sorrel King to present what happened to Josie at a conference of healthcare professionals so that they could hear her story. She talked about the need for parents to be allowed to call in emergency response teams when their hospitalized child might be in danger. She said that if she had been able to activate a team like this, she believes that Josie would still be alive and that other families whose children have died from medical errors might also have been able to avoid their tragic losses. As a result of her idea, two hospitals in Pittsburgh initiated a program of rapid response that could be activated by a concerned family and that brings a team of physician, nurse, respiratory therapist, and patient safety officer to a child's bedside. The program was called Condition H, where *H* stands for help. The family-initiated rapid response team program has since spread to hospitals throughout the nation as a patient safety initiative to improve the quality of care delivery.

A new public-private partnership, the Partnership for Patients: Better Care, Lower Costs, was launched to improve the quality, safety, and affordability of health care. This partnership brings together hospital leaders, employers, clinicians, patient advocates and officials from state and federal governments to improve quality. It has two primary goals: (1) to keep patients safe from injury and getting sicker by reducing preventable, hospital-acquired conditions by 40% before 2014, and (2) to help patients recover and heal free from complications by preventing complications when patients transition to another care setting and to decrease readmissions by 30% (http://www.healthcare.org). As an advocate for this partnership, Sorrel King continues to speak to health professionals and tell them the Josie King story. In addition to creating the website for the Josie King foundation (http://www.josieking.org), she has authored a book to reach additional audiences called *Josie's Story*. Her memoir is a heartening effort to make sure health practitioners remember that when even one preventable death occurs, one is too many.

DISCUSSION QUESTIONS:

1. In what ways did ineffective communication contribute to Josie's death?

2. Carry out a root cause analysis using a fishbone diagram to identify all the possible contributing causes in the preventable death of Josie King. What category has the most contributing factors: people, processes, equipment, environment, management, or regulation?

3. How might a culture of blame perpetuate safety problems and affect morale among clinicians?

4. Would the hospital's response in this situation help the clinicians cope with the feelings of grief and guilt that they might have experienced?

5. Apply the PDSA rapid cycle change process to Condition H using the Model for Improvement questions and identifying the plan, do, study, act parts of the change cycle as if you were going to consider trying Condition H in your organization.

References

American Association of Colleges of Nursing. (2011). *The essentials of master's education in nursing.* Washington, DC: Author.

Blendon, R. (2011). *America's views on the quality of healthcare.* Retrieved from http://www.hsph.harvard.edu/news/press-releases/poll-us-health-care-quality/

Deming, W. E. (1986). *Out of the crisis.* Cambridge, MA: MIT Center for Advanced Engineering Study.

Donabedian, A. (1980). *Exploration in quality assessment and monitoring, Vol. I: The definition of quality and approaches to its assessment.* Ann Arbor, MI: Health Administration Press.

Finkelman, C., & Kenner, C. (2010). *Professional nursing concepts: Competencies for quality leadership.* Sudbury, MA: Jones and Bartlett.

Gerteis, M., Edgman-Levetan, S., & Daley, J. (1993). *Through the patient's eyes. Understanding and promoting patient-centered care.* San Francisco, CA: Jossey-Bass.

Harris Interactive. (2010, December 2). *The Harris Poll #149.* Retrieved from http://www.prnewswire.com/news-releases/oil-pharmaceutical-health-insurance-and-tobacco-top-the-list-of-industries-that-people-think-should-be-more-regulated-111183714.html

Hassmiller, S. (2012). About. Retrieved from http://www.thefutureofnursing.org/about/

Institute of Medicine. (1999). *To err is human: Building a safer health system.* Washington, DC: National Academy Press.

Institute of Medicine. (2001). *Crossing the quality chasm: A new health system for the 21st century.* Washington, DC: National Academy Press.

Institute of Medicine. (2007). *Preventing medication errors: Quality chasm series.* Washington, DC: National Academy Press.

Ishikawa, K. (1987). *Guide to quality control* (trans. Asian Productivity Organization). White Plains, NY: Kraus International Publications.

Joint Commission. (2003). *Sentinel event alert.* Retrieved from http://www.jointcommission.org/sentinel_event_alert_issue_28_infection_control_related_sentinel_events/

King, S. (2002). Sorrel's speech to IHI conference. Presented at Institute for Healthcare Improvement National Conference. Retrieved from http://www.josieking.org/whathappened

Langley, G. L., Nolan, K. M., Nolan, T. W., Norman, C. L., & Provost, L. P. (2009). *The improvement guide: A practical guide to enhancing organizational performance.* San Francisco, CA: Jossey-Bass.

National Research Council (2003). *Health professions education: A bridge to quality.* Washington, DC: The National Academies Press.

Schyve, P. (2005). Systems thinking and patient safety. In K. Henriksen, J. Battles, E. Marks, & D. Lewin (Eds.), *Advances in patient safety: From research to implementation* (Vol. 2, pp. 1–4). Rockville, MD: Agency for Healthcare Research and Quality.

Spath, P. (2009). *Introduction to healthcare quality management.* Chicago, IL: Health Administration Press.

Youngberg, B. J., & Weber, D. R. (1997). Integrating risk management, utilization management, and quality management: Maximizing benefit through integration. In C. G. Meisenheimer (Ed.), *Improving quality: A guide to effective programs (2nd ed.).* Gaithersburg, MD: Aspen Publishers.

CHAPTER 7

Health Policy and Advocacy: Practice to the Full Extent

Mary Virden, RN, MSEd

Learning Objectives

At the completion of this chapter, you will be able to:

1. Explain the importance of recognizing predictable patterns in managing change.
2. List five types of patient data a practice might use to support patient care.
3. Describe common barriers to access to care.
4. List eight key areas or critical domains of transformation to a patient-centered medical home.
5. Understand the financial implications of the patient-centered medical home.
6. Compare the traditional medical model to the patient-centered model of care.

This chapter examines what can be described as the epitome of professional nursing practice, in which delivery of care means patients receive well-coordinated services and enhanced access to a clinical team. At the time this case begins, consensus of what constitutes a "medical home" was still developing, and there was scant peer-reviewed literature on the efficacy of the medical home model. Now it is commonly accepted that clinicians practicing in a patient-centered medical home (PCMH) use decision support tools, measure their performance, engage patients in the patients' own care, and conduct quality improvement activities to address patients' needs. This case also illustrates the potential of the PCMH model to increase clinical quality, improve patient experience, and reduce health system costs.

Part I: Background

NURSING PRACTICE IN KANSAS

This case occurs in Kansas, where regulations governing advanced nursing practice authorize each Advanced Practice Registered Nurse (APRN) to make independent decisions about needs of families, patients, and clients and medical decisions. This regulation does not require the immediate and physical presence of a physician when care is given by the APRN. Each APRN is directly accountable and responsible to the consumer, developing and managing the medical plan of care for patients based upon an annually reviewed collaborative practice agreement developed jointly by the APRN and one or more physicians (Kansas State Board of Nursing, 2013).

DEMOGRAPHIC BACKGROUND

Metropolitan Wyandotte County (Kansas City, Kansas) is the fourth most densely populated urban county in Kansas, with a 2010 U.S. Census estimated total population of 157,505. Unemployment is high (10.3% in 2009); thus, the median household income is low at $37,316. (By comparison, the Kansas median household income is $47,709.) More than 21% of county residents have incomes below the federal poverty level, making Wyandotte County one of the poorest counties in the state of Kansas.

Wyandotte is a federally recognized low-income population Health Professional Shortage Area (HPSA) and state-designated Medically Underserved Area (MUA).

The U.S. Census Bureau 2011 American Community Survey projected the percentage of uninsured individuals in Wyandotte younger than age 65 years to be 22.9%, compared to 15.8% statewide. There are estimated to be 15,702 Medicare beneficiaries in WyCo age 65 and older.

Estimates of racial and ethnic population distribution in 2011 were 54.6% White, 25.2% Black or African American, 26.4% Hispanic (any race), and very small percentages of American Indian/Alaskan Natives, Asians, and Native Hawaiian/Other Pacific Islanders.

Education levels in Wyandotte are also among the lowest in Kansas. According to the U.S. Census Bureau 2010 American Community Survey, 21% of the county population had less than a high school education. When stratified by race and ethnicity, the lack of education becomes even more pronounced; almost 24% of African Americans and more than 56% of Hispanics in the county had less than a high school education.

Silver City Health Center (SCHC) was a private physician's practice in the Argentine community within Wyandotte County that was acquired by KU Medical Center in 1997 and managed for 9 years by the School of Medicine as a residency program training site. In July 2006, management was transferred to KU HealthPartners, the faculty practice plan for the Schools of Nursing and Health Professions. SCHC is currently the only academically affiliated, nurse-run safety net clinic in Kansas. Leadership of the clinic consists of a master's-prepared clinic director and four family practice and one pediatric APRNs. This case chronicles the 5-year journey from private medical practice to a nationally recognized medical home.

Part II: Practice Transformation: Where to Begin?

In 2006, when community members were asked their impressions of Silver City Health Center, most were conflicted about their feelings. "I like that the clinic is in our neighborhood, but I don't ever see the same doctor." "I used to get medication for my diabetes there, but then the special program ended." Through an interpreter, "They don't have very many people who speak my language." Disappointment with continuity and access was rampant throughout the community.

As a residency program training site, the clinic was staffed mainly by nonprofessionals (front office staff and medical assistants) and a part-time registered nurse. Staff was accustomed to telephones being answered and first appointments beginning at 9:00 a.m., a 1.5-hour lunch period during which the door was locked and phones went unanswered, and a closing time with phone rollover at 4:00 p.m. The clinic's priorities were resident physician training, clinical trials research, and patient care.

MODEL OF CARE DEVELOPMENT

Although the term *patient-centered medical home* was not prevalent in 2006, the necessity for change was obvious to the master's-prepared nurse leadership team. Student training is certainly important and research is integral to the academic environment; however, prioritizing patient care third seemed inverted. But where to begin, and what route would lead to success with such a wholesale transformation of culture and practice systems? Could a strategy of engaged leadership, coupled with quality improvement, develop the fundamental base required to enable SCHC to learn and implement change?

Nurse leaders were familiar with two organizations with published core concepts related to placing the patient at the center of health care: the Picker Institute, with its Principles of Patient Centered Care (http://www.pickerinstitute.org/), and the American Academy of Family Physicians' TransforMed Project (http://www.transformed.com/). Based on knowledge of the work of both groups, SCHC nurse leaders began to develop the foundation for their model of care (**Figure 7-1**).

During a 2-day staff retreat, all staff members contributed to creating examples of what each of the eight domains of SCHC's model of care might mean to patients. For instance, staff felt

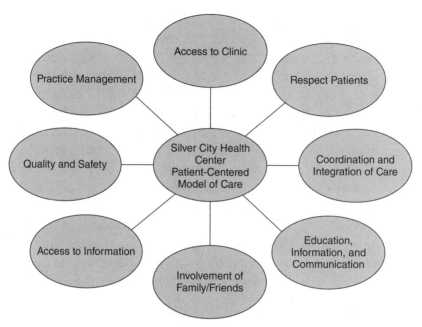

FIGURE 7-1 SCHC Model of Care, based upon Picker Institute's Patient-Centered Care Model and AAFP's TransforMED.
Source: Reprinted with permission by KU HealthPartners, Inc.

"access to clinic" might include routine, urgent care, and walk-in appointment availability; waiting time once a patient is in the clinic; how and when the phones are answered; hours of operation and after-hours availability; the physical environment, including decorating, cleanliness, and pediatric safety; language barriers; and external and internal signage.

CHANGES DRIVEN BY THE MODEL OF CARE

Aspects of this model became the lead-off discussion at each subsequent monthly staff meeting, with staff members prompted by leadership to recognize other staff with public kudos, when they were "caught in the act" of patient-centered excellence in a model domain. Because staff members had all contributed to developing the model, with consistent repetition over time this discussion became an ingrained "way of being," and staff members were overheard acknowledging others without reminder.

Additionally, this focus on patient-centered care became the basis for a difficult culture change within SCHC. Staff who had traditionally gone out to lunch together were now required to stagger their shifts. This provided access for patients during the lunch hour, when employed patients who don't have a phone available during the work day could contact the clinic. During the staff meeting when this change was being deliberated, the front office supervisor was vehemently and vocally opposed, saying, "*My* doctor doesn't stay open over the lunch hour!" To which a medical assistant replied, "Yes, but don't you wish he did?" Progress is measured in small steps!

Finally, discussion of the quality and safety and access domains of SCHC's model of care rapidly contributed to a realization that the historical clinic location was unacceptably undersized, dilapidated, and without essentials of clinical care, such as running water in each exam room, which nurse leaders expected of a high-quality, patient-centered practice. Therefore, within 8 months of assuming management of SCHC, KU HealthPartners located an alternative site in the Argentine community, negotiated a multiyear lease, renovated the new site, and relocated the clinic.

DISCUSSION QUESTIONS

1. Think about your state. Are advanced practice nurses required to have a physician physically on site? If so, how might the role of the master's-prepared nurse in this practice site differ from that in a nurse-run practice? What potential benefits and challenges might you encounter with this practice model as you think about developing a medical home?

2. Do your organization's goals and vision include explicit language about becoming a patient-centered medical home? Why or why not?

3. Do you agree that engaged leadership and a quality improvement strategy are foundational requirements in creating a medical home? Why or why not?

Part III: Building Relationships

Practice leadership recognized that interactions among and between staff, providers, patients, patient families, and the community were a critical predictor of success or failure in establishing a medical home. Without strong internal team relationships, leadership felt the push for patient-centeredness would be initially well received but eventually short-lived. Therefore, team building within the practice was an early and sustained focus.

INTERNAL TEAMBUILDING

In the beginning, relationships among "inherited" staff members and the new nurse practitioner providers and nurse leaders needed a great deal of nurturing. Teambuilding within the practice required a constant commitment to questioning, listening, helping, sharing, and building trust. Nurse leaders acknowledged the crucial importance of ongoing, open communication, strong vision for change, and relentless follow-through to lead the team toward success.

Social science researchers have long documented that each group of people has a distinct personality. Nurse leaders knew that staff members, themselves included, fall somewhere within a bell curve of the following categories when confronting change: innovators, early adopters, early majority, late majority, and laggards (Rogers, 2003). Many change efforts founder because of leaders' concentration on the laggards, who see high risk in adopting a new idea, challenge leaders' thinking, and cause the team to "bog down." SCHC's practice leaders chose to focus on the early adopters and early majority who were able to make the connection between the new ideas and their personal needs and were willing to serve as a test laboratory while the leaders worked out the bugs and revised plans to reach SCHC's goals. Staff members and providers in these groups looked for simple, proven, better ways of doing their jobs. Many who were initially skeptical of the changes were brought on board as they observed success and wanted to follow.

Unfortunately, some of those in the tiny group of laggards began to negatively influence other staff members with their fears and opinions. Although prudence required SCHC nurse leadership to listen carefully to this small group, eventually these staff members were invited to "get on board" or assisted to find another position that was better suited to their needs and desires. In retrospect, being able to say, "Where we want to go with SCHC no longer appears to be a match for where you want to go and how you want to work," enabled a painful parting of the ways to be completed honestly and respectfully. It was extremely helpful to remember the adage "The only one who truly likes change is a wet baby!"

PATIENT AND COMMUNITY RELATIONSHIPS

Concurrently with internal team building, it was clear that relationships with patients and their families as well as with the broader Argentine community needed to be repaired and nurtured. Positive patient interactions are transmitted rapidly by word of mouth within the Hispanic community, where more than 60% of SCHC patients live. In addition, increased and ongoing connections with other local healthcare-related, government, and civic organizations allowed nurse leaders to actively participate in community activities, more accurately assess community needs, and positively influence others' perceptions of SCHC.

Building strong, long-term relationships or continuity of care between patients and their providers fosters improved communication, trust, and knowledge of patient backgrounds and preferences. SCHC began to focus on developing and/or revising position descriptions for all staff to include roles and responsibilities associated with the medical home, hiring professionals and nonprofessionals who met these expanded criteria, and reorganizing care so that it could be provided by a team of professionals and specially trained nonprofessionals, rather than by a single individual provider.

EMPANELMENT

These changes all helped SCHC establish and provide organizational support for care delivery teams that are accountable for the patient population. Increased knowledge of patients and their needs provided support for linking patients to a provider and care team in a process called "empanelment." Pairing patients and a provider care team enabled them to recognize each other as partners in care.

Empanelment required SCHC to first ensure that all patients were assigned a primary care provider through a clearly defined process. Because the population of patients served by SCHC is ethnically and racially diverse with numerous social determinants of health, establishing appropriate and equitable panel sizes for each provider required SCHC to identify patient acuities, adjusting not only for the medical complexity of the patient but also for social determinants of care.

Unable to discover evidence-based tools for ascertaining ambulatory acuities in a safety net population, nurse leaders created their own tool, which included not only chronic illnesses and medications but also language spoken by the patient, health literacy and social needs, self-management ability, and mental health (**Figure 7-2**). Additional supports for this new empanelment approach included new procedures, such as a means for patients who wanted to change their provider assignment; development, ongoing review, and revision of policies addressing provider productivity and scheduling; continuous review and adjustment of provider and nonprofessional staffing; and a script for front office staff to use for patient appointment scheduling. Continuing periodic review of provider panels provided SCHC with improved abilities to effectively judge staffing levels and scheduling needs and address provider orientation, workload equity, and other concerns, thus increasing the likelihood of productive interactions between patients and care teams.

Part IV: Changing Care Delivery

It is not enough to create more efficient business structures or provide greater access to care without ensuring care is based upon current scientific evidence and is well planned and organized. SCHC's APRNs were eager to improve the care they offered through measuring, benchmarking, and improving clinical performance and patient interactions.

FIGURE 7-2 SCHC Patient Acuity Rubric.

PATIENT ACUITY RUBRIC

Please select the criteria number from the drop-down menu next to the category name. For example, if your patient has a steady income or stable residency you would select a zero next to the category name "social".

Patient Name: ___ (insert name)

Provider: ___ (insert name)

DOB: ___ (enter patient DOB) _____

Evaluation Date: ___ (enter date of evaluation) _____

CATEGORY		CRITERIA		
		0	1	2
Social Please select which criteria your patient falls under next to the category name "social"	0	• Steady income • Independent • Stable residency • Family or other support system • Adequate medical insurance coverage	• Able to meet some of social needs with help of family/others or some form of income • Some medical insurance coverage	• Requires multiple provider interventions for social situation • Minimal to no resources available for social needs • Completely dependent on others for basic social needs • No insurance coverage
Language Please select which criteria your patient falls under next to the category name "language"	0	• Consistent with provider	• Some ability to communicate in provider's language	• Needs interpreter for all interactions with provider
Health Literacy Please select which criteria your patient falls under next to the category name "health literacy"	0	• Appropriate demonstration of understanding of healthcare needs • Explores health information independently	• Moderate understanding of healthcare needs • Requires some routine provider reinforcement	• Demonstrates minimal understanding of healthcare needs • Requires routine reinforcement and explanation
Ability to Self Manage Please select which criteria your patient falls under next to the category name "ability to self manage"	0	• Minimal provider intervention to carry out plan of care • Demonstrates self-management (example: blood sugar log presented each visit with appropriate home testing regimen)	• Somewhat able to carry out plan of care • Requires some provider intervention and reinforcement	• Repeated provider reinforcement and intervention required

Source: Reprinted with permission by KU HealthPartners, Inc.

CATEGORY	CRITERIA 0	CRITERIA 1	CRITERIA 2
Mental Health Please select which criteria your patient falls under next to the category name "mental health"	• No mental health issues <u>or</u> • Long-term stability demonstrated	• Has mental health issues but is under the routine care of a mental health care provider • Requires some provider intervention	• Has mental health issues not adequately controlled • Multiple and repeated provider intervention and support
Chronic Illnesses Please select which criteria your patient falls under next to the category name "chronic illnesses"	• No chronic illnesses <u>or</u> • Long-term stability demonstrated	• Has chronic illness(es), which • Requires some provider intervention (i.e. specialist referrals, frequent monitoring, etc.)	• Has chronic illness(es) not adequately controlled • Multiple and repeated provider intervention and support
Chronic Medications 0 Please select which criteria your patient falls under next to the category name "chronic medications"	• No chronic illnesses <u>or</u> • Long-term stability demonstrated	• Has chronic illness(es), which • Requires some provider intervention (i.e. specialist referrals, frequent monitoring, etc.)	• Has chronic illness(es) not adequately controlled • Multiple and repeated provider intervention and support
Comments:			

Category	Score
Social	0
Language	0
Health Literacy	0
Self-Management	0
Mental Health	0
Chronic Illnesses	0
Chronic Meds	0
TOTAL	0

Interpretation of Total Score

Point Range	Acuity	Category
0 - 4	LOW	A
5 - 9	MEDIUM	B
> or = 9	HIGH	C
Patient's Acuity Category		0

DISCUSSION QUESTIONS

1. How can visible and sustained leadership contribute to overall culture change?

2. Read the following statements:

   No one will make changes if they do not understand the need to do so; they cannot make changes without ideas as to what they might do differently; and they certainly cannot transform their organization without effective strategies for implementation.

   Do you agree? Why or why not?

3. How does thinking of a whole population of patients, as well as individual patients, differ from the traditional medical model of care? What implications might a population focus have in the structure of the practice or in delivery of care?

4. What are the advantages of using care delivery teams? Are there disadvantages to this model?

CHRONIC CARE MODEL

The Chronic Care Model (CCM) served as a guide to SCHC providers who initially focused on improving care for diabetic patients. This model summarizes the basic elements for improving care for chronically ill individuals and populations (**Figure 7-3**) (Improving Chronic Illness Care, 2013). Each of the six elements of the model is important individually, but the elements also interact with and support each other. SCHC targeted three key areas for improvement efforts as the practice gained more experience: planned care, decision support, and care management.

Planned care, deliberately designed to ensure that patient needs are met (1) identifies essential clinical tasks associated with evidence-based care (e.g., performing a comprehensive diabetic foot assessment), (2) identifies who on the team should perform the task, (3) reviews patient data prior to the visit to identify needed services, and (4) structures the encounter so that relevant team members can deliver all needed services, assisted by standing orders and other protocols. By 2007, while considering

The Chronic Care Model

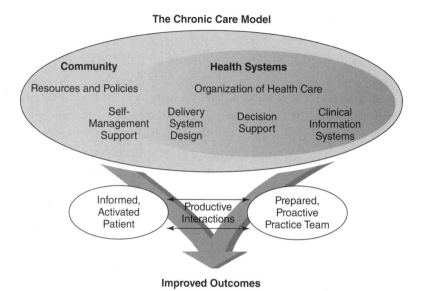

Improved Outcomes

FIGURE 7-3 Chronic Care Model, developed by the MacColl Institute.
Source: Reproduced from Wagner E. H. (1998). Chronic disease management: What
will it take to improve care for chronic illness? *Effective Clinical Practice, 1*, 2–4.

planned care for diabetic patients, nurse leaders recognized that
the addition of a dietitian and a physical therapist to the care team
would facilitate an interprofessional, team-based comprehensive
approach to diabetic care, improve low rates of nutrition counseling and annual comprehensive foot evaluation, and potentially
decrease high rates of lower extremity-related complications. Subsequent analysis of data showed positive clinical outcomes for
SCHC's population of diabetic patients (Peterson & Virden, 2012).

Decision support increases the likelihood that care adheres to
evidence-based guidelines. Although SCHC did not use an electronic medical record to assist providers in making appropriate
clinical decisions for diabetic patients, the practice recognized
the utility of a chronic disease registry and paper-based tools to
increase the visibility of evidence-based clinical guidelines and
make them easier for providers and care teams to follow.

Finally, in 2009 SCHC began to provide *care management
services* for diabetic patients. These services included identifying
patients who had not been seen in a defined period of time and
assisting them to schedule appointments, providing information

and counseling to help patients set goals and develop action plans to more effectively self-manage their health, and providing care coordination to help integrate care when patients needed services from other providers or agencies. This closed-loop approach to coordinating care ensures that the care team is involved and assisting a patient at every step, from the time the provider recommends other services, until the patient has an appointment and is seen, the specialist's report is received back by SCHC, and the care team or provider communicates results and has developed a plan for next steps with the patient.

ELECTRONIC SUPPORT FOR CARE DELIVERY

Use of the chronic disease registry allowed SCHC providers to periodically review clinical data for the diabetic population. Improving trends in clinical metrics, such as the percentage of patients with hemoglobin A1c levels at or below 7.0% and the percentage of diabetic patients who had more than two encounters in the previous year, reinforced the conviction that improvement in care was possible (**Figure 7-4**). This contributed to a decision to expand the programmatic approach to delivery of chronic care, from a focus solely on diabetic patients to include all patients with hypertension and hyperlipidemia.

Concurrently with the maturation of data reliability in the chronic disease registry, the experience with reporting capabilities allowed more sophisticated and reliable reports. Leaders and providers also began to better utilize already-collected data in SCHC's practice management system. Moreover, nurse leaders discovered the practice management system had the capacity to be tailored to report data that had not previously been considered important. Finally, the benefits of electronic support for care led to use of a statewide immunization registry. This was originally implemented solely in 2006 for recording and reporting pediatric immunizations, but was adopted by 2008 for all immunizations administered in the practice. In combination, the chronic disease registry, practice management system, and immunization registry formed a backbone of electronic support in a paper-based chart environment.

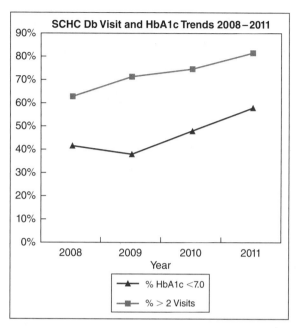

FIGURE 7-4 SCHC Diabetes Quality of Care Metrics.
Source: Reprinted with permission by KU HealthPartners, Inc.

MEASURING PATIENT INTERACTIONS

In addition to "hard data," SCHC leaders believed the "voice of the patient" was needed to effectively respond to patients' values and preferences and to improve their experience of care. Routine feedback from patients and families was solicited often, clarified, communicated widely throughout the practice, and, most important, acted upon. This approach required a respect for patients' values and expressed needs that took some staff members time to develop because it was perceived by some as negating "the good care we have always given." However, seeking answers to questions in various ways (written surveys, point-of-care data collection, patient and family walk-throughs) combined with an inquisitive approach to the discovery of information provided real help in planning changes and reinforced improvements in care delivery. Although patients may not know whether SCHC providers offered evidence-based, quality care, they do know whether their provider gave them information that was helpful, whether they feel better, or whether they or their families know what to do in case of emergency.

The importance of setting realistic expectations for the amount of time and effort needed to see results when collecting patient experience data was a significant lesson learned. The pace of change and improvement can be time-consuming and dauntingly slow. Nonetheless, SCHC leaders found that involving patients early in the process of designing new materials, for example, by soliciting their input, was exciting for the patients and gave staff confidence that was formerly lacking when changes were contemplated.

DISCUSSION QUESTIONS

1. How does the use of data contribute to the ability to support patient care for individual patients? For a population of patients?
2. What could the concepts of planned care and decision support mean in your setting?
3. How might putting patients and families on your improvement team help achieve success in transformation?

Part V: Reducing Barriers

Over time, SCHC leaders and providers acknowledged that other essential improvements were required if the practice was to become truly patient-centered. Although no less important than previous progress, improving access to care and reducing care fragmentation were not occurring as quickly or as seamlessly as desired.

IMPROVING ACCESS TO CARE

A key element of access to care is ensuring patients have 24/7 continuous access to their care teams. During office hours, developing expectations for staff and providers and communicating to patients how quickly phone messages would be returned proved no more difficult to implement than were many other changes. However, addressing after-hours access was challenging. APRNs who had not previously had on-call responsibilities were now accountable for developing a call schedule, documenting after-hours patient advice, and communicating patient calls to the patients' primary care providers. These changes required true dedication on the part of nurse clinicians to "keeping the patient in the center," and, in a world of paper charts, this meant new processes and procedures deliberately designed to effectively support simplified communication.

Another element of access to care is determining patient preferences regarding clinic hours of operation. As SCHC began to solicit this information from patients, the practice moved toward expanding appointment availability; current hours changed to 7:00 a.m. to 5:00 p.m. 3 days per week and 7:00 a.m. to 7:00 p.m. 2 days. Additional evening services such as smoking cessation classes and a Teen Clinic have also been evaluated.

Lack of insurance also contributed to limited access to care for many. Wyandotte County has a large immigrant population, many of whom are not eligible for public insurance. However, many families in SCHC's patient population have parents and older children who are not eligible for public insurance, but younger children who are. Their parents either do not know how or are afraid to access the state system for eligibility determination. Thus, an agreement with a state agency was developed that placed an eligibility determination worker on site 3 days per week, greatly increasing the number of children who had Medicaid insurance and assisting the practice to more rapidly determine adult patients' eligibility.

REDUCING FRAGMENTATION

The complex "system" of care delivery is frequently nonnavigable and frustrating for patients in the safety net environment, especially those who have a different cultural background, may not have insurance, may not speak English, and may not have knowledgeable family support. Obtaining specialty services for the uninsured or for those on Medicaid is particularly difficult. Reducing fragmentation through effective care coordination for all patients, not just those with diabetes, became an ongoing goal for SCHC.

Nurse leaders developed numerous written agreements with community agencies and specialty providers to facilitate referrals and respond to social service needs. In 2007, SCHC began to use an e-referral system to facilitate information transfer to enable specialists to have the clinical data they needed at the time of a patient's visit. Tracking and supporting patients when they obtain services outside SCHC became a service for all. A process to communicate test results and care plans to patients and families was also initiated, supported by written procedures and routine effectiveness monitoring. Following up with patients within a few days of emergency department use or hospitalization was aided by a closer relationship between SCHC and the primary referring hospital. However, the cost of staffing to provide care management services for high-risk patients and integration of behavioral health and specialty care into SCHC care delivery has proven to be problematic.

DISCUSSION QUESTIONS

1. What benefits or outcomes might be associated with improved access to care for the following:
   a. Patients and families
   b. Providers
   c. Clinics
   d. Communities
2. Why is care coordination so difficult?
3. Why might patients use the emergency department as a source of nonurgent care? Why should patients, providers, and payers have an interest in reducing the number of avoidable emergency department visits?

Conclusion

In early 2011, Silver City Health Center was recognized by the National Committee for Quality Assurance (NCQA) as a Level 3 Patient-Centered Medical Home (PCMH), the first public or private clinic in Kansas to achieve this designation.

Payer and policymaker enthusiasm for the PCMH model of care stems from the belief that a practice that provides high-quality primary care will improve outcomes and reduce healthcare costs by meeting patient needs for accessible, continuous, comprehensive, coordinated services and planned, evidence-based, patient-centered care. This belief was validated by SCHC's improved continuity of care, access to care, clinical and patient experience outcomes, and decreased systemwide costs.

IMPROVING OUTCOMES

Continuity of care outcomes are measured by tracking the number and percentage of patients empaneled (assigned to a primary care provider) and the percentage of primary care visits patients have with their assigned primary care provider. Since empanelment was implemented in early 2010, continuity percentages across the practice have increased from 78% to an average of 89%, with several individual practitioners averaging more than 92%. No-show rates (the percentage of patients with scheduled appointments who do not keep them and do not call prior to the appointment to cancel or reschedule) practice-wide have dropped from 37% in 2009 to 12% in 2012.

Access to care is tracked and trended by measuring the number of days to "third next available" appointment by provider and across both adult and pediatric service areas. In 2008, the average number of days to third next available appointment for adults averaged more than 20 days. By late 2011, the average was 4 to 6 days. Wait times for pediatric appointments were never lengthy and continue to average 1 to 2 days to third next available appointment. The "third next available" appointment is used rather than the "next available" appointment because it is a more sensitive reflection of true appointment availability. For example, an appointment may be open at the time of a request because of a cancellation or other unexpected event. Using the third next available appointment eliminates such chance occurrences from the measure of availability (Institute for Healthcare Improvement, n.d.).

Clinical outcomes data illustrate improving quality of care for SCHC patients with diabetes over the years 2008 to 2010, during which time the number of patients with diabetes tracked in the electronic chronic disease management system increased by 30% from 157 to 211. The percentage of patients with hemoglobin A1c (HbA1c) levels < 7.0% improved from less than 40% to more than 58%, and those who had more than two visits in a year increased from slightly more than 60% to more than 80% (**Figure 7-4**). Similar progress was seen in hypertension metrics in the same time period: the percentage of patients with controlled hypertension (blood pressure < 130 and < 80 mm Hg) increased from 28% to more than 47% (**Figure 7-5**). Additionally, reports from the immunization registry confirmed a dramatically improved pediatric immunization rate. SCHC was also recognized in 2010 by the Kansas Department of Health and Environment as one of the top two clinics in the state for HPV immunizations.

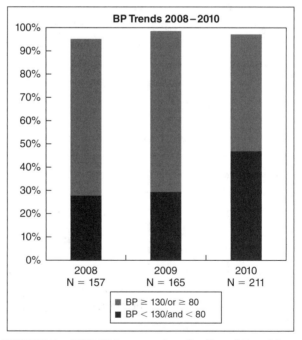

FIGURE 7-5 SCHC Hypertension Quality of Care Metrics.
Source: Reprinted with permission by KU HealthPartners, Inc.

Patient experience metrics likewise demonstrate a high level of satisfaction with medical home domains of access to care, communication with their provider and staff members, coordination of care, and whole person care. More than 97% of those responding say SCHC is their regular source of care, and 98% state they would refer family and friends to SCHC.

FINANCIAL IMPLICATIONS

Nurse leaders believed there was a systemwide return on investment, achievable by establishing a patient-centered medical home and care coordination for those who need follow-up to hospital care and who do not have a routine healthcare provider. In early 2012, SCHC concluded an 18-month quality improvement study of the utilization of service and cost of uncompensated care for 55 adult patients who established a medical home following referral from the University of Kansas Hospital, SCHC's primary source of new patients. An analysis of these patients' utilization in the 365 days prior to establishing care at Silver City showed 14 inpatient stays with an average length of stay of 3.9 days and 76 emergency department visits. In the year after establishing care with Silver City, these 55 patients had 4 inpatient stays with an average length of stay of 1.5 days and 19 emergency department visits (**Figure 7-6**).

The systemwide financial implications of SCHC's medical home were striking. In the 12 months after these patients established with SCHC, the cost of their uncompensated care in the emergency department dropped from $190,364 to $18,314. Inpatient costs declined from $300,114 to less than $1,000. The average uncompensated cost per patient declined from $5,450 to $1,408, for a systemwide cost reduction of 84.2%. The potential systemwide cost savings of the medical home model of care were more than $5.2 million in avoided costs, if extrapolated to the entire adult population at SCHC. If these savings were coupled with potential cost avoidance for approximately 180 new community adult patients who directly establish a medical home at SCHC annually, the potential avoided costs would be even higher.

Outcomes: Reduced KUMC Systemwide Uncompensated Care Costs

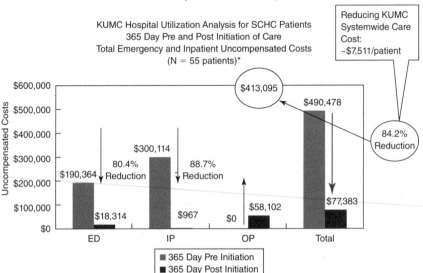

* At the end of FY-11, SCHC Patient Panel = 704 adults × $7,511 saved per patient in first year = $5,287,744 in avoided hospital costs.

* Note: Hospital Utilization data provided by KUH Care Management, Organizational Improvement and Patient Financial Services Departments. Analysis includes patients with a 1st Date of Service at SCHC on or before 10/26/10 with hospital utilization data through 10/26/11.

FIGURE 7-6   SCHC Uncompensated Care Outcomes.
Source: Reprinted with permission by KU HealthPartners, Inc.

CHANGE CONCEPTS

The wholesale transformation of SCHC's practice entailed an extensive variety of small changes in many different aspects of the organization. The practice was assisted in its medical home design by a local foundation, which financially supported training and a consultant to assist with implementation of NCQA PCMH standards. This consultation helped SCHC practice leaders recognize that there was order in the chaos of transformation. The majority of the interrelated changes could be broadly grouped into eight conceptual categories: (1) engaged leadership; (2) quality improvement strategy; (3) empanelment; (4) continuous, team-based healing relationships; (5) patient-centered interactions; (6) organized, evidence-based care; (7) enhanced access; and (8) care coordination (Safety Net Medical Home Initiative, 2014).

As SCHC gained experience, many of the changes associated with these broad categories felt natural, but others required a great deal of study and experimentation to tailor the concept to SCHC.

Although not specifically addressed in this case, the importance of leadership dedicated to administration and a comprehensive view of the organization was a significant factor in achievement of PCMH designation. It is very difficult for APRNs who are focused on daily patient care to also dedicate thought and time to the executive and management needs of the medical home. Having a committed administrative leader was an invaluable aid to transformation.

The journey continues, as nurse leaders are aware that formal recognition provides only a snapshot of a longer quality improvement voyage toward development and implementation of excellence in clinical service through innovative practice models, with emphasis on strategies for sustaining change and leadership opportunities for master's-prepared nurses.

References

Improving Chronic Illness Care. (2013). Our approach. Retrieved from http://www.improvingchroniccare.org/

Institute for Healthcare Improvement. (n.d.). Third next available appointment. Retrieved from http://www.ihi.org/resources/Pages/Measures/ThirdNextAvailableAppointment.aspx

Kansas State Board of Nursing. (2013). Kansas Nurse Practice Act. Retrieved from http://www.ksbn.org/npa/npa.pdf

Peterson, J. M., & Virden, M. D. (2012). Improving diabetic foot care in a nurse-managed safety-net clinic. *Journal of the American Academy of Nurse Practitioners, 25*(5), 263–271. doi:10.1111/j.1745–7599.2012.00786.x

Rogers, E. M. (2003). *Diffusion of innovations*. New York, NY: Free Press.

Safety Net Medical Home Initiative. (2014). Patient-centered care for the safety net. Retrieved from http://www.safetynetmedicalhome.org/change-concepts/

CHAPTER 8

Patient Safety: Congressional Action

Angela S. Mattie, JD, MPH

Learning Objectives

At the completion of this chapter, you will be able to:

1. Gain knowledge of the legislative process and its impact on healthcare organizations.
2. Understand the role of advocacy organizations in shaping healthcare policy.
3. Realize the significance of patient safety issues to the healthcare field.
4. Define organizations involved in patient safety.

Background

On July 29, 2005, President Bush signed into law the Patient Safety Quality Improvement Act (P.L. No. 109-41). This long-awaited bill came after significant debate in the Senate and the House.

The Institute of Medicine's 1999 landmark report, *To Err Is Human: Building a Safer Health System*, brought the significance of patient safety issues to the national forefront and called for congressional action. The Institute of Medicine (IOM) reported that healthcare errors represent the eight leading cause of death in the United States (Centers for Disease Control and Prevention [CDC], 1999). Estimates indicate that between 44,000 and 98,000 Americans die each year as a result of medical errors (American Hospital Association, 1999). More people die each year as a result of medical errors than from motor vehicle accidents (43,458), breast cancer (42,297), or AIDS (16,516) (CDC, 1999).

The costs to the healthcare system and economy are significant. National costs as a result of medical errors are estimated at between $17 billion and $29 billion (Thomas et al., 1999). If other industries lived with the same failure rate, we would have two unsafe landings per day at O'Hare, 16,000 pieces of mail lost every hour, and 32,000 bank checks deducted from the wrong bank account every hour (Leape, 1994).

One emerging theme from the IOM report is something that Donald Berwick, a medical doctor, first articulated in a 1988 publication: that "there are no bad apples, just bad systems"(Berwick, 1989). The IOM report recognized that doctors, nurses, and healthcare workers are human, humans are prone to errors, and when errors occur they are mostly likely attributed to system failures.

Several recommendations emerged from the IOM report. Those recommendations where congressional action was required included: (1) the establishment of a national Center for Patient Safety in the Agency for Health Care Research and Quality (AHRQ); (2) the creation of a national, state-based mandatory reporting system for adverse events that result in serious injury or death with public disclosure of these events; (3) the development of voluntary reporting systems to generate information on healthcare errors, especially near misses/close calls, and system flaws with protection against disclosure of reported information; and (4) the passage of legislation to extend peer review protections to data related to patient safety and quality improvement that are collected and analyzed by healthcare organizations for internal use or shared with others solely for purposes of improving safety and quality (Institute of Medicine [IOM], 1999).

The Institute of Medicine followed *To Err Is Human* with several other reports focusing on healthcare quality. For example, *Crossing the Quality Chasm: A New Health System for the 21st Century* (IOM, 2001a) identifies gaps in the delivery of patient care services and articulates the need for leadership to facilitate change, commit to a statement of purpose, and adopt a new set of principles to foster patient safety. *Envisioning a National Health Care Quality Report* (IOM, 2001b) addresses the collection, measurement, and analysis of quality data.

The IOM, recognizing the critical role of nurses in patient safety, produced a 2003 report: *Keeping Patients Safe: Transforming the Work Environment for Nurses.* This report called for immediate reforms to the systems in which nurses work. These reforms included increasing nursing staff, placing limits on the numbers of hours that a staff nurse may work, and once again calling for a medical error and near miss reporting system. Emphasized was the need for this system to have whistleblower protections to shield reporters of medical errors from retaliation.

Yet despite the significant monetary and mortality costs associated with medical errors, it was 6 years after the first IOM report before Congress passed legislation in this area. A dialogue on this issue began on Capitol Hill shortly after the 1999 Institute of Medicine report, *To Err Is Human: Building a Safer Health System.* The U.S. Senate Health, Education, Labor, and Pensions (HELP) committee has held numerous hearings on this issue. Each congressional session since the 105th Congress has produced some version of patient safety legislation. However, passage was thwarted partly because of disagreement and conflicting arguments on what role Congress should play and what were the fundamental principles required in federal patient safety legislation.

This text explores the development of patient safety legislation through the use of a class exercise highlighting the competing stakeholders' positions, an analysis of the major issues requiring resolution and compromise prior to bill passage, and finally use of an actual case resulting in criminal conviction for nurses. This final section illustrates the potential impact patient safety legislation can have on changing the "culture of blame and shame" into a culture that promotes a nonpunitive, learning environment that leads to significant improvements in healthcare quality.

Analyzing Different Views

Most lawmakers would be hard pressed to argue with the policy behind the Patient Safety and Quality Improvement Act: to encourage safer practices in our hospitals and healthcare facilities. Then, why did passage of this bill take so long? A partial answer requires understanding of the importance of interest groups and their influence on Capitol Hill. The old adage that you do not want to see laws or sausage made certainly applies to the development of the Patient Safety and Quality Improvement Act. Interest groups and advocacy organizations play a significant role in influencing the development of healthcare legislation. Although agreement may have existed on the basic premise of improving patient safety, much debate occurred around the principles to be incorporated in the bill.

Healthcare lobbying plays an important and influential role in the development of healthcare legislation. Healthcare associations, their lobbyists, and other stakeholders such as the trial lawyers all weighed in on the issue of patient safety. Frequent Capitol Hill visits, the development of position statements, mobilization of grassroots efforts, and meetings occurred on this issue. Lobbyists often bring their position on a particular bill directly to the senators, members of Congress, and/or their staff. Associations often draft position statements on behalf of their members and disseminate this information through their websites. Grassroots efforts are mobilized to support these positions. Association members are urged to contact their member of Congress and state their position. For example, the American Medical Association (AMA) is sophisticated in mobilizing grassroots efforts on healthcare issues, often posting sample letters, talking points, and congressional addresses on its website.

Significant lobbying efforts were devoted to arguing and attempting to find agreement on the basic principles to be incorporated in a patient safety bill. Although there are no specific data on lobbying expenditures allocated to supporting competing positions for patient safety legislation, lobbying expenditures focused on healthcare issues totaled $237 million in 2000. These expenditures accounted for 15% of all federal lobbying and were larger than the lobbying expenditures of every other sector, including agriculture, communications, and defense. A total of 1,192 organizations were involved in healthcare lobbying (Landers & Sehgal, 2004).

CLASS EXERCISE: UNDERSTANDING ADVOCACY ORGANIZATIONS' INFLUENCE ON HEALTHCARE POLICY

Students should review the websites of the American Association for Justice (formerly the Association of Trial Lawyers of America; http://www.justice.org/cps/rde/xchg/justice/hs.xsl/default.htm/), the American Nurses Association (http://www.ana.org/), and the Leapfrog Group (http://www.leapfroggroup.org/) in preparation for this exercise.

Numerous advocacy organizations played an active and vocal role in the development of patient safety legislation. Understanding these organizations' different perspectives is important to comprehending the complexity of the legislative process. This exercise is designed to highlight the different and often competing perspectives. Three associations are used for this illustration: The American Association for Justice was very active in representing the views of plaintiffs and plaintiffs' attorneys. The American Nurses Association (ANA) was selected to illustrate healthcare providers' views and perspectives. The Leapfrog Group was selected to highlight the views of employers, who have come to recognize the importance of being involved in healthcare policy debates.

American Association for Justice

The American Association for Justice is a well-funded, sophisticated organization that played an important role in the political process surrounding patient safety legislation. Trial lawyers by profession rely on adversarial dispute resolution in health care. As the world's largest trial bar, the American Association for Justice promotes justice and fairness for injured persons, safeguards victims' rights, and strengthens the civil justice system through education and disclosure of information critical to public health and safety (http://www.justice.org/cps/rde/xchg/justice/hs.xsl/about.htm).

DISCUSSION QUESTIONS

Assume you are the legislative director for the American Association for Justice.

1. What principles would you want incorporated in the patient safety bill?
2. Which one of these principles would you most strongly lobby?
3. Why would this be important?

American Nurses Association

ANA also maintains a strong presence on Capitol Hill. Dedicated to ensuring that an adequate supply of highly skilled and well-educated nurses is available, ANA is committed to meeting the needs of nurses as well as healthcare consumers. ANA advances the nursing profession by fostering high standards of nursing practice, promoting the economic and general welfare of nurses in the workplace, projecting a positive and realistic view of nursing, and lobbying Congress and regulatory agencies on healthcare issues that affect nurses and the general public.

DISCUSSION QUESTIONS

You have been asked to draft a position statement for ANA on patient safety.

1. What key principles would the nursing profession desire to include in this position statement?
2. Why are these principles important to your profession?

Leapfrog Group

Healthcare expenditures represent 14.8% of the gross domestic product. A significant part of these expenditures is borne by U.S. employers. Until recently, employers have played a passive role in assessing and analyzing how their healthcare benefit dollars are spent. Realizing the impact employers as large purchasers of health care could have on healthcare quality and affordability, a group of employers formed the Leapfrog Group. The 1999 IOM report served as a major impetus for this group's formation. *To Err Is Human* recommended that large employers provide market reinforcement for the quality and safety of health care. The Leapfrog Group is composed of more than 170 companies and organizations that purchase health care.

The mission of this organization is to reduce preventable medical mistakes and improve the quality and affordability of health care; encourage public reporting of healthcare quality and outcomes so that consumers and purchasing organizations can make more informed healthcare choices; reward doctors and hospitals for improving the quality, safety, and affordability of health care; and help consumers reap the benefits of making smart healthcare decisions.

DISCUSSION QUESTIONS

1. What role, if any, should the Leapfrog Group play in the patient safety debate on Capitol Hill?

2. Why is it important for employer groups to be involved in this debate?

3. What principles should this organization support in the formation of patient safety legislation?

The different perspectives of trial lawyers, providers, and employers needed resolve prior to agreement on the major principles to be contained in patient safety legislation. Lobbying efforts of these and other organizations played a major role in the final legislation. The following section outlines major areas of conflict and solutions reached during the numerous years of debate on this legislation.

The Major Issues

LEGAL AND CONFIDENTIALITY PROTECTIONS FOR PATIENT SAFETY DATA: THE MAIN ISSUE

One of the major controversies surrounding the development and passage of patient safety legislation focused on whether patient safety data should be afforded legal and confidentiality protections. The 1999 IOM report specifically recommended:

> Congress should pass legislation to extend peer review
> protections to data related to patient safety and quality
> improvement that are collected and analyzed by health care
> organizations for internal use or shared with others solely for
> purposes of improving safety and quality. (IOM, 1999, p. 10)

The IOM recognized that an important component of a comprehensive strategy to improve patient safety is to create an environment that encourages organizations to identify errors, evaluate causes, and design systems to prevent future errors from occurring. This could not be achieved without specific legal protections for those data collected through patient safety activities.

Following the IOM report, the U.S. Senate committee on Health, Education, Labor, and Pensions (HELP), which has jurisdiction over health policy matters, held no fewer than five hearings focusing on patient safety. Through these hearings, the committee found that efforts to improve patient safety required creating a learning environment characterized by supportive, voluntary data-gathering systems. Testimony of experts such as Tommy Thompson, secretary of the Department of Health and Human Services, and Donald Berwick, a medical doctor and nationally known healthcare quality expert, agreed with the research in this field, calling for the creation of a "safe harbor" for the reporting of medical error information; that is, a means of reporting and analyzing information insulated from the risk of incurring additional liability (U.S. Senate Committee on Health, Education, Labor, and Pensions, 2003).

Advocacy organizations such as the American Medical Association strongly favored legal and confidentiality protections for data generated through patient safety activities, whereas the American Association for Justice was strongly opposed to such protections. As the advocacy organizations articulated their position on Capitol Hill, they illuminated the existing tension between the tort system and patient safety principles. The powerful and well-seasoned lobbying efforts representing both sides of this debate were perhaps the major factor in slowing the passage of patient safety legislation.

The primary goals of tort liability for medical malpractice are to compensate injured patients, deter negligence, and dispense corrective justice. However, healthcare quality experts argued that the current tort system "undercuts the evolution of an effective safety culture in health care institutions" (Bovbjerg & Raymond, 2003). An effective culture of patient safety requires an atmosphere of learning, feedback, and improvement. Although not the only reason, fear of retribution and litigation often impedes creating a culture of safety, analyzing errors, and seeking and implementing opportunities for improvement.

Peer review does offer a process for physicians and healthcare providers to analyze performance of their colleagues and to evaluate and improve care. All states, with the exception of New Jersey, have enacted laws that protect the proceedings of peer review committees from discovery in the legal process. The courts, however, in recent years appear to be piercing the confidentiality protections afforded to these peer review activities and narrowly construing the confidentiality protections in favor of discovery. For example, in a medical malpractice claim against a hospital where a patient had accidentally been disconnected from a ventilator, the court allowed the discovery of incident reports submitted to a hospital peer review committee as well as recommendations for corrective action of the committee (*Chicago Trust Co. v. Cook County Hosp.*, 1998).

Therefore, for patient safety legislation to be truly effective, that is, to encourage reporting, analysis of errors, and design of improvements in care, it would require federal protections for the confidentiality of the data reported. Not surprisingly, the American Association for Justice lobbied fiercely against these protections because it feared that these protections would provide hospitals and healthcare providers with a mechanism to shield information on medical errors from discovery and the legal process. Additionally, there is a growing consumer movement calling for the public release of healthcare data.

A compromise was needed that both sides could accept. When a medical error occurs, it is most likely a result of a system failure, not an aberrant healthcare provider. Hospital and healthcare facilities must be free to seek opportunities for improvement.

What is required in most instances is a root cause analysis of the event. Root cause analysis (RCA) is a methodology employed by healthcare facilities and practitioners to identify the "root cause" or actual reason or reasons for the incident. Data gathering is usually the first step in conducting an RCA. During this phase, the process for care may be flow-charted, or data can be gathered by other methods. The focus of this methodology is to identify what, how, and why something happened to design and implement improvements to prevent further reoccurrences. Conducting a root cause analysis necessitates reviewing processes of care and continually asking why an event occurred. Details of the event are generated and solutions developed to avoid future issues. The healthcare community must be free to explore improvements without fear that these data will be used in the legal process. This nonpunitive environment is necessary to promote a culture of safety.

A balance was required between the need to allow plaintiffs to seek redress through the tort system of medical practice liability and the need to promote a learning environment for continuous quality improvement. After much debate on this issue, the bill that was signed into law accomplishes this balance.

Confidentiality protections apply only to those data and work products generated as a result of a patient safety event or near miss and submitted to patient safety organizations (PSOs). In other words, the legal and confidentiality protections apply only to the Patient Safety Work Product (PSWP). PSWP is defined in the legislation as any data, reports, records, memoranda, analyses (such as root cause analyses), or written or oral statements that: (1) are assembled or developed by a provider for reporting to a PSO and are reported to the PSO or (2) are developed by a PSO for the conduct of patient safety activities (Patient Safety and Quality Improvement Act, 2005). PSWP also includes work product that identifies or constitutes the deliberations and analysis of the event.

The intent is that the PSO will take this information and provide feedback to avoid future occurrences. Healthcare facilities will be free to investigate the event and design opportunities for improvement without the fear that information will result in a legal process. Plaintiffs and their attorneys will still have the ability to use the legal system to obtain medical records, billing, discharge information, or any other original patient or provider record. The confidentiality protections do not extend backward to the event, but only serve to encourage a complete and open investigation to identify the root cause of the issue and make this information available to other healthcare facilities.

The act further provides that PSWP is privileged and may not be: (1) subject to subpoenas, orders, or discovery request issued in a federal, state, or local civil or criminal case; (2) subject to disclosure under the Freedom of Information Act or any similar state or local law; (3) admitted as evidence in any governmental proceeding; or (4) admitted in any professional or disciplinary proceeding (Patient Safety and Quality Improvement, 2005).

MANDATORY VERSUS VOLUNTARY REPORTING OF MEDICAL ERRORS

Another issue of much debate was whether the patient safety reporting requirements should be mandatory or voluntary. The IOM report recommended a mandatory reporting system for adverse events that result in death or serious harm (IOM, 1999, p. 9). At the same time, the IOM also recommended that voluntary reporting efforts be encouraged (IOM, 1999, p. 9).

Mandatory reporting systems are most often operated by regulatory agencies that have investigatory authority. These systems focus on serious or sentinel events in which the patient is seriously harmed. The underlying principle for most of these systems is to protect society from harm. Opponents to mandatory systems state that they are limited in their ability to capture information on less severe events or near misses and complete information on more serious events (Agency for Healthcare Research and Quality, 2003). Healthcare entities often fear retribution, and this promotes a culture of blame.

Proponents of voluntary reporting systems argue that voluntary reporting systems are key to creating improvements in healthcare quality. Confidential, nonpunitive systems encourage identification of potential problems, full disclosure of system issues, and an analysis of the underlying system problems.

During testimony presented at congressional hearings on patient safety, representatives from the Department of Veterans Affairs (VA) articulated the requirement to establish a voluntary, nonpunitive system of reporting medical errors and near misses. The VA is generally recognized as a leader in patient safety. Established in 1999, the VA's National Center for Patient Safety takes a systems approach to improving patient safety based on prevention, not punishment. Once an event is reported to the VA system, quality improvement tools are employed to identify the root causes of the event or potential event and solutions are designed and implemented. On an annualized basis, the VA saw a 30-fold increase in reporting of adverse events and a 900-fold increase in reporting of close calls (U.S. Senate Committee on Health, Education, Labor, and Pension, 2001).

Congress apparently incorporated the advice of patient safety experts from the VA and used the successful history of other industries such as the Federal Aviation Administration (FAA) when drafting the Patient Safety and Quality Improvement Act of 2005. The FAA's Aviation Safety Reporting System (ASRS) encourages airline personnel to voluntarily report incidents in which aviation safety is compromised. The ASRS analyzes the submitted incident reports to identify discrepancies so corrective action can be taken.

The resulting legislation encourages healthcare providers to voluntarily report medical errors to patient safety organizations.

WHISTLEBLOWER PROTECTIONS: THE NEED TO PROTECT THE REPORTER

Closely tied to the call for confidentiality and legal protections for patient safety data was the need for reporter protections for healthcare providers who identify and report events to a patient safety organization (PSO). ANA and others lobbied strongly for whistleblower protections for those reporting patient safety events. It is widely recognized that one of the major impediments to reporting is physicians', nurses', and other healthcare professionals' fear about job security and the use of reports in disciplinary and adverse employment actions.

Proponents of reporter protections argued that if a reporting system is to be truly effective, that is, result in real improvements in quality of care, then those who report events must be free of the fear of retaliation. In 2004, while enacting a patient safety reporting statute, the New Jersey legislature noted the major problem in underreporting: "fear of sanctions induces health care professionals and organizations to be silent about adverse events, resulting in serious under-reporting" (N.J. Stat. Ann., 2005).

The Patient Safety and Quality Improvement Act of 2005 includes reporter protections. The bill provides that a provider may not take an adverse employment action against an individual based on the fact that the individual in good faith reported information either to a provider with the intent of having that information reported to a PSO or directly to a PSO. This protection also applies to adverse evaluations or decisions made in relation to accreditation, certification, credentialing, or licensing of the individual.

STATES' REPORTING SYSTEMS: WHAT ROLE FOR THE FEDERAL GOVERNMENT?

Before patient safety legislation could become a reality yet another issue required resolution: What should the relationship of this federal legislation be with states' patient safety statutes and/or regulations? State legislatures acted more quickly than did the federal government in the area of establishing reporting systems for patient safety. Twenty-four states passed legislation or regulations related to hospital reporting of adverse events. Of these, 23 states required mandatory reporting of adverse events and 1 implemented a voluntary system. (California, Colorado, Connecticut, Florida, Georgia, Kansas, Illinois, Massachusetts, Maryland, Maine, Minnesota, Nevada, New York, New Jersey, Ohio, Oregon, Pennsylvania, Rhode Island, South Carolina, South Dakota, Tennessee, Texas, Utah, and Washington. Oregon is the only voluntary system. Massachusetts has two mandatory reporting systems.) The majority of states created systems that are based on the IOM's recommendation for mandatory reporting systems. Many states include both accountability and a learning component in their systems. In the majority of states, the overriding purpose for these systems is to hold healthcare entities accountable for performance.

Some states attempt to emphasize the learning component of these systems by distributing safety alerts when incidents with significant consequences are reported.

Other states attempt to aggregate the data they collect to identify patterns and trends across facilities.

However, states are limited in their ability to use the data generated by these systems to make real improvements in patient safety. An October 2005 report published by the National Academy for State Health Policy noted:

> States may be challenged by small numbers of reportable and/or reported events, lack of resources, and lack of clinical expertise, all of which may limit states' ability to produce reliable trend data and identify best practices. In addition, state reporting systems are in various stages of implementation and many are in the process of determining how best to analyze and share information with reporting facilities. (Rosenthal & Booth, 2005)

Despite the challenges inherent in states' reporting systems, controversy over the role the federal government should play in this arena still existed. The eventual legislation established a floor for certain protections applicable to the Patient Safety Work Product (PSWP) and does not limit or preempt the application of other federal, state, or local laws that provide greater privilege or confidentiality protections. This legislation also does not preempt state laws that require providers to report information that is not PSWP.

PATIENT SAFETY ORGANIZATION: WHO SHOULD ASSUME THE ROLE?

Patient safety organizations are responsible for collecting, analyzing, and providing recommendations on information submitted on patient safety events. Two issues existed concerning the role of patient safety organizations. The first issue was how patient safety organizations should be organized: Should they be a central site or should multiple organizations assume the role? The second issue was how patient safety organizations should be established in a way that would enhance and not intercept the current work in the public and private arenas.

When examining the organizational issue, the IOM report and Congress looked to other industries with successful reporting systems. In particular, the FAA's Aviation Safety Reporting System (ASRS) was considered as a model for an effective reporting system. The FAA's ASRS consists of one national database located at a central site. It receives about 30,000 reports annually and has an operating budget of approximately $2 million. It was estimated that 1 million errors occur each year in the hospital setting, and this figure did not account for the significant number of close calls. Congress concluded that a centralized site for reporting errors would be "prohibitively expensive and impractical. Not only would the sheer number of reports be overwhelming, but also the necessary expertise that would be required to properly analyze reports would be prohibitive" (U.S. Senate Committee on Health, Education, Labor, and Pensions, 2003).

The preferred approach was to take a "let the flowers bloom" mentality. Although not explicitly stated, this philosophy would gain for the bill advocates from already existing systems rather than opponents from entities fearing loss of their systems. In addition, this approach would build on the numerous public and private activities.

Several national systems already existed. As previously discussed, almost half the states have some type of reporting system. In addition, many private initiatives were under way. For example, The Joint Commission, an independent, nonprofit organization responsible for accrediting hospitals and healthcare organizations, has in place a sentinel events reporting system. The Joint Commission defines a sentinel event as one that results in an unanticipated death or major permanent loss of function not related to the natural course of the patient's illness or underlying condition. The Joint Commission does not take adverse action against the healthcare entity's accreditation status for reporting sentinel events. This system was in place since 1996. Not surprisingly,

The Joint Commission maintained a strong presence on the Hill during the debates on the patient safety bill.

Several other private initiatives focused on medication error reporting. For example, since 1975 the Institute for Safe Medication Practices (ISMP) had in place a Medication Errors Reporting System. Practitioners report medication errors and near errors to this reporting system. The ISMP publishes biweekly reports and special alerts. This information makes the healthcare industry aware of such events as lookalike or sound-alike drugs, dosage issues, route of administration issues, and so forth.

Under the new law, all existing public and private entities will have the option of applying for certification as a patient safety organization. The patient safety bill establishes fairly stringent criteria for entity certification as a patient safety organization. Among other requirements, to qualify for certification entities must have appropriately trained staff, the mission and primary activity of conducting activities to improve patient safety and the quality of healthcare delivery, and the purpose of providing direct feedback and assistance to providers to effectively minimize patient risk. An organization seeking to become a PSO must submit an initial certification to the secretary of the Department of Health and Human Services, and this certification must be renewed every 3 years.

ELECTION YEAR 2004: PATIENT SAFETY A PERIPHERAL ISSUE

Another impediment to passage focused primarily on politics rather than policy: Activity on this legislation took a back seat to the 2004 presidential election. At the time of the election, both the House and the Senate had passed patient safety legislation. Minor differences existed between the two versions of the bill. The Senate-approved bill had stronger provisions to protect health professionals who report medical errors from retaliation by their employers. The House-approved bill had stronger provisions guarding against conflict of interest on the part of PSOs and more stringent requirements for the certification of PSOs. These issues alone did not account for the increased length of time for the bill passage. More likely, it was the role potential passage of this bill played in the presidential election. It took a back seat to more pressing issues, such as the war in Iraq, the budget deficit, and in the healthcare arena the cost of prescription drugs.

CASE STUDY: *Does the Patient Safety and Quality Improvement Act of 2005 Accomplish Its Goal?*

In July 2005, the Patient Safety and Quality Improvement Act of 2005 was sent to President Bush for his signature and became Public Law 109-41. This chapter has discussed the major issues and the role advocacy organizations played in the development of this legislation. Following is a case that occurred before implementation of this law and a discussion of what might happen under Public Law 109-41.

BEFORE IMPLEMENTATION OF PSQIA: A CULTURE OF BLAME

In 1996, in Colorado an infant died as a result of a medication error. A physician had ordered a single, intramuscular dose of penicillin; a hospital pharmacist mistakenly sent to the unit a much larger dose. The neonatal nurse changed the medication to intravenous to avoid sticking the child repeatedly with such a large dose. Three registered nurses were charged with criminally negligent homicide. Two nurses pleaded guilty and received 2 years of probation and 24 hours of public service. The third nurse was acquitted.

AFTER IMPLEMENTATION OF PSQIA: A NONPUNITIVE, LEARNING ENVIRONMENT

If this case had occurred after the Patient Safety and Quality Improvement Act of 2005 became a law, the hospital would have been free to conduct a root cause analysis to discover the system errors that resulted in this tragic event. The root cause analysis, information discovered, and changes and improvements in the system implemented as a result of this quality investigation would have become patient safety work product as defined in the legislation. These data would have been afforded the confidentiality and legal protections contained in the law and therefore would be shielded from discovery and other legal proceedings. The hospital would have been free from the fear of litigation as a result of its diligence in investigating the event and designing solutions to prevent future occurrences. The nurses and other healthcare providers who reported this event to a patient safety organization would have received the protection of the "whistleblower" provision in the legislation. These reporters would have been protected from any adverse employment action resulting from reporting.

The patient safety organization would have analyzed data submitted from this occurrence and, if appropriate, would have aggregated them with data from other such events. Any global issues and conclusions would have been widely disseminated to the healthcare community with solutions to advert this event from occurring elsewhere.

The patient's family would still have recourse available through the tort system and could pursue medical malpractice litigation. Medical records, insurance information, and admission and discharge notes would still be available for discovery in these legal proceedings. Data generated from this event in an attempt to discover the system error and implement corrections to ensure no subsequent events follow would be protected.

Conclusion

The Patient Safety and Quality Improvement Act fosters an environment in which providers are encouraged to learn from mistakes that result from poor systems and to make corrections to those systems to improve the quality of care delivered. As Neil Armstrong said upon taking his first step on the moon: "That's one small step for a man, one giant leap for mankind." The Patient Safety and Quality Improvement Act was a long time in coming. The confidentiality and legal protections are a small step toward changing the healthcare environment from a punitive approach to errors to one that seeks the opportunity for improvement, but this small step is a giant leap for changing the culture and improving the quality of care delivered in healthcare facilities.

References

Agency for Healthcare Research and Quality. (2003, December). AHRQ's Patient Safety Initiative: Building foundations, reducing risk. Interim report to the Senate Committee on Appropriations. Retrieved from http://www.ahrq.gov/research/findings/final-reports/pscongrpt/index.html

American Hospital Association. (1999). *Hospital statistics.* Chicago, IL: Author.

Berwick, D. M. (1989). Continuous improvement as an ideal in health care. *New England Journal of Medicine, 320,* 53–56.

Bovbjerg, R. R., & Raymond, B. (2003, January). *Patient safety, just compensation and medical liability reform.* Oakland, CA: Kaiser Permanente. Retrieved from http://www.kpihp.org/wp-content/uploads/2012/12/patient_safety.pdf

Centers for Disease Control and Prevention, National Center for Health Statistics. (1999). Births and deaths: Preliminary data for 1998. *National Vital Statistics Reports, 47*(25), 6.

Chicago Trust Co. v. Cook County Hosp., 698 N.E. 2d 641 (Ill. App. Ct. 1998).

Institute of Medicine. (1999). *To err is human: Building a safer health system.* Washington, DC: National Academy Press.

Institute of Medicine. (2001a). *Crossing the quality chasm: A new health system for the 21st century.* Washington, DC: National Academy Press.

Institute of Medicine. (2001b). *Envisioning a national health care quality report.* Washington, DC: National Academy Press.

Institute of Medicine. (2003). *Keeping patients safe: Transforming the work environment for nurses.* Washington, DC: National Academy Press.

Landers, S. H., & Sehgal, A. R. (2004). Health care lobbying in the United States. *American Journal of Medicine, 116*(7), 474–477.

Leape, L. L. (1994). Error in medicine. *Journal of the American Medical Association, 272*(23),1851–1857.

N.J. Stat. Ann. & 26:2H-12.24(e) (2005).

Patient Safety and Quality Improvement Act of 2005, Pub. L. No. 109-41.

Rosenthal, J., & Booth, M. (2005). *Maximizing the use of state adverse event data to improve patient safety.* Washington, DC: National Academy for State Health Policy.

Thomas, E. J., Studdert, D. M., Newhouse, J. P., Zbar, B. I., Howard, K. M., Williams, E. J., & Brennan, T. A. (1999). Costs of medical injuries in Utah and Colorado. *Inquiry, 36*, 255–264.

U.S. Senate Committee on Health, Education, Labor, and Pensions. (2001, May 25). Hearing on patient safety: What is the role for Congress? Testimony of Dr. Jim Bagian.

U.S. Senate Committee on Health, Education, Labor, and Pensions. (2003). Patient Safety and Quality Improvement Act of 2003, S. Rep. No. 108-196 (2003).

Appendix A: Public Law 109-41: The Patient Safety and Quality Improvement Act of 2005

UNITED STATES PUBLIC LAWS
109th Congress—1st Session
(c) 2005, LEXIS-NEXIS, A DIVISION OF REED ELSEVIER INC. AND REED ELSEVIER PROPERTIES INC.
PUBLIC LAW 109-41 [S. 544]
JUL. 29, 2005
109 P.L. 41; 119 Stat. 424; 2005 Enacted S. 544; 109 Enacted S. 544

BILL TRACKING REPORT: 109 Bill Tracking S. 544
FULL TEXT VERSION(S) OF BILL: 109 S. 544
An Act
To amend title IX of the Public Health Service Act to provide for the improvement of patient safety and to reduce the incidence of events that adversely effect patient safety.

Be it enacted by the Senate and House of Representatives of the United States of America in Congress assembled,

[*1] SECTION 1. SHORT TITLE; TABLE OF CONTENTS.

(a) Short Title.—This Act may be cited as the "Patient Safety and Quality Improvement Act of 2005".
(b) Table of Contents.—The table of contents for this Act is as follows:

[*2] SEC. 2. AMENDMENTS TO PUBLIC HEALTH SERVICE ACT.

(a) In General.—Title IX of the Public Health Service Act (42 U.S.C. 299 et seq.) is amended—
    (1) in section 912(c), by inserting", in accordance with part C," after "The Director shall";
    (2) by redesignating part C as part D;
    (3) by redesignating sections 921 through 928, as sections 931 through 938, respectively;
    (4) in section 938(1) (as so redesignated), by striking "921" and inserting "931"; and
    (5) by inserting after part B the following:

C "PART C—PATIENT SAFETY IMPROVEMENT

"Sec. 921. DEFINITIONS.

"In this part:

"(1) HIPAA confidentiality regulations.—The term 'HIPAA confidentiality regulations' means regulations promulgated under section 264(c) of the Health Insurance Portability and Accountability Act of 1996 (Public Law 104-191; 110 Stat. 2033).

"(2) Identifiable patient safety work product.—The term 'identifiable patient safety work product' means patient safety work product that—

"(A) is presented in a form and manner that allows the identification of any provider that is a subject of the work product, or any providers that participate in activities that are a subject of the work product;

"(B) constitutes individually identifiable health information as that term is defined in the HIPAA confidentiality regulations; or

"(C) is presented in a form and manner that allows the identification of an individual who reported information in the manner specified in section 922(e).

"(3) Nonidentifiable patient safety work product.—The term 'nonidentifiable patient safety work product' means patient safety work product that is not identifiable patient safety work product (as defined in paragraph (2)).

"(4) Patient safety organization.—The term 'patient safety organization' means a private or public entity or component thereof that is listed by the Secretary pursuant to section 924(d).

"(5) Patient safety activities.—The term 'patient safety activities' means the following activities:

"(A) Efforts to improve patient safety and the quality of health care delivery.

"(B) The collection and analysis of patient safety work product.

"(C) The development and dissemination of information with respect to improving patient safety, such as recommendations, protocols, or information regarding best practices.

"(D) The utilization of patient safety work product for the purposes of encouraging a culture of safety and of providing feedback and assistance to effectively minimize patient risk.

"(E) The maintenance of procedures to preserve confidentiality with respect to patient safety work product.

"(F) The provision of appropriate security measures with respect to patient safety work product.

"(G) The utilization of qualified staff.

"(H) Activities related to the operation of a patient safety evaluation system and to the provision of feedback to participants in a patient safety evaluation system.

"(6) Patient safety evaluation system.—The term 'patient safety evaluation system' means the collection, management, or analysis of information for reporting to or by a patient safety organization.

"(7) Patient safety work product.—

"(A) In general.—Except as provided in subparagraph (B), the term 'patient safety work product' means any data, reports, records, memoranda, analyses (such as root cause analyses), or written or oral statements—

"(i) which—

"(I) are assembled or developed by a provider for reporting to a patient safety organization and are reported to a patient safety organization; or

"(II) are developed by a patient safety organization for the conduct of patient safety activities; and which could result in improved patient safety, health care quality, or health care outcomes; or

"(ii) which identify or constitute the deliberations or analysis of, or identify the fact of reporting pursuant to, a patient safety evaluation system.

"(B) Clarification.—

"(i) Information described in subparagraph (A) does not include a patient's medical record, billing and discharge information, or any other original patient or provider record.

"(ii) Information described in subparagraph (A) does not include information that is collected, maintained, or developed separately, or exists separately, from a patient safety evaluation system. Such separate information or a copy thereof reported to a patient safety organization shall not by reason of its reporting be considered patient safety work product.

"(iii) Nothing in this part shall be construed to limit—

"(I) the discovery of or admissibility of information described in this subparagraph in a criminal, civil, or administrative proceeding;

"(II) the reporting of information described in this subparagraph to a Federal, State, or local governmental agency for public health surveillance, investigation, or other public health purposes or health oversight purposes; or

"(III) a provider's recordkeeping obligation with respect to information described in this subparagraph under Federal, State, or local law.

"(8) Provider.—The term 'provider' means—

"(A) an individual or entity licensed or otherwise authorized under State law to provide health care services, including—

"(i) a hospital, nursing facility, comprehensive outpatient rehabilitation facility, home health agency, hospice program, renal dialysis facility, ambulatory surgical center, pharmacy, physician or health care practitioner's office, long term care facility, behavior health residential treatment facility, clinical laboratory, or health center; or

"(ii) a physician, physician assistant, nurse practitioner, clinical nurse specialist, certified registered nurse anesthetist, certified nurse midwife, psychologist, certified social worker, registered dietitian or nutrition professional, physical or occupational therapist, pharmacist, or other individual health care practitioner; or
"(B) any other individual or entity specified in regulations promulgated by the Secretary.

"SEC. 922. PRIVILEGE AND CONFIDENTIALITY PROTECTIONS.

"(a) Privilege.—Notwithstanding any other provision of Federal, State, or local law, and subject to subsection (c), patient safety work product shall be privileged and shall not be-

"(1) subject to a Federal, State, or local civil, criminal, or administrative subpoena or order, including in a Federal, State, or local civil or administrative disciplinary proceeding against a provider;

"(2) subject to discovery in connection with a Federal, State, or local civil, criminal, or administrative proceeding, including in a Federal, State, or local civil or administrative disciplinary proceeding against a provider;

"(3) subject to disclosure pursuant to section 552 of title 5, United States Code (commonly known as the Freedom of Information Act) or any other similar Federal, State, or local law;

"(4) admitted as evidence in any Federal, State, or local governmental civil proceeding, criminal proceeding, administrative rulemaking proceeding, or administrative adjudicatory proceeding, including any such proceeding against a provider; or

"(5) admitted in a professional disciplinary proceeding of a professional disciplinary body established or specifically authorized under State law.

"(b) Confidentiality of Patient Safety Work Product.—
Notwithstanding any other provision of Federal, State, or
local law, and subject to subsection (c), patient safety work
product shall be confidential and shall not be disclosed.

"(c) Exceptions.—Except as provided in subsection (g)(3)—

"(1) Exceptions from privilege and confidentiality.—
Subsections (a) and (b) shall not apply to (and shall not
be construed to prohibit) one or more of the following
disclosures:

"(A) Disclosure of relevant patient safety work
product for use in a criminal proceeding, but only
after a court makes an in camera determination
that such patient safety work product contains
evidence of a criminal act and that such patient
safety work product is material to the proceeding
and not reasonably available from any other
source.

"(B) Disclosure of patient safety work product to the
extent required to carry out subsection (f)(4)(A).

"(C) Disclosure of identifiable patient safety work
product if authorized by each provider identified in
such work product.

"(2) Exceptions from confidentiality.—Subsection
(b) shall not apply to (and shall not be construed to
prohibit) one or more of the following disclosures:

"(A) Disclosure of patient safety work product to
carry out patient safety activities.

"(B) Disclosure of nonidentifiable patient safety
work product.

"(C) Disclosure of patient safety work product to
grantees, contractors, or other entities carrying
out research, evaluation, or demonstration
projects authorized, funded, certified, or otherwise
sanctioned by rule or other means by the Secretary,
for the purpose of conducting research to the extent
that disclosure of protected health information
would be allowed for such purpose under the
HIPAA confidentiality regulations.

"(D) Disclosure by a provider to the Food and Drug Administration with respect to a product or activity regulated by the Food and Drug Administration.

"(E) Voluntary disclosure of patient safety work product by a provider to an accrediting body that accredits that provider.

"(F) Disclosures that the Secretary may determine, by rule or other means, are necessary for business operations and are consistent with the goals of this part.

"(G) Disclosure of patient safety work product to law enforcement authorities relating to the commission of a crime (or to an event reasonably believed to be a crime) if the person making the disclosure believes, reasonably under the circumstances, that the patient safety work product that is disclosed is necessary for criminal law enforcement purposes.

"(H) With respect to a person other than a patient safety organization, the disclosure of patient safety work product that does not include materials that—

"(i) assess the quality of care of an identifiable provider; or

"(ii) describe or pertain to one or more actions or failures to act by an identifiable provider.

"(3) Exception from privilege.—Subsection (a) shall not apply to (and shall not be construed to prohibit) voluntary disclosure of nonidentifiable patient safety work product.

"(d) Continued Protection of Information After Disclosure.—

"(1) In general.—Patient safety work product that is disclosed under subsection (c) shall continue to be privileged and confidential as provided for in subsections (a) and (b), and such disclosure shall not be treated as a waiver of privilege or confidentiality, and the privileged and confidential nature of such work product shall also apply to such work product in the possession or control of a person to whom such work product was disclosed.

"(2) Exception.—Notwithstanding paragraph (1), and subject to paragraph (3)—

"(A) if patient safety work product is disclosed in a criminal proceeding, the confidentiality protections provided for in subsection (b) shall no longer apply to the work product so disclosed; and

"(B) if patient safety work product is disclosed as provided for in subsection (c)(2)(B) (relating to disclosure of nonidentifiable patient safety work product), the privilege and confidentiality protections provided for in subsections (a) and (b) shall no longer apply to such work product.

"(3) Construction.—Paragraph (2) shall not be construed as terminating or limiting the privilege or confidentiality protections provided for in subsection (a) or (b) with respect to patient safety work product other than the specific patient safety work product disclosed as provided for in subsection (c).

"(4) Limitations on actions.—

"(A) Patient safety organizations.—

"(i) In general.—A patient safety organization shall not be compelled to disclose information collected or developed under this part whether or not such information is patient safety work product unless such information is identified, is not patient safety work product, and is not reasonably available from another source.

"(ii) Nonapplication.—The limitation contained in clause (i) shall not apply in an action against a patient safety organization or with respect to disclosures pursuant to subsection (c)(1).

"(B) Providers.—An accrediting body shall not take an accrediting action against a provider based on the good faith participation of the provider in the collection, development, reporting, or maintenance of patient safety work product in accordance with this part. An accrediting body may not require a provider to reveal its communications with any patient safety organization established in accordance with this part.

"(e) Reporter Protection.—

"(1) In general.—A provider may not take an adverse employment action, as described in paragraph (2), against an individual based upon the fact that the individual in good faith reported information—

"(A) to the provider with the intention of having the information reported to a patient safety organization; or

"(B) directly to a patient safety organization.

"(2) Adverse employment action.—For purposes of this subsection, an 'adverse employment action' includes—

"(A) loss of employment, the failure to promote an individual, or the failure to provide any other employment-related benefit for which the individual would otherwise be eligible; or

"(B) an adverse evaluation or decision made in relation to accreditation, certification, credentialing, or licensing of the individual.

"(f) Enforcement.—

"(1) Civil monetary penalty.—Subject to paragraphs (2) and (3), a person who discloses identifiable patient safety work product in knowing or reckless violation of subsection (b) shall be subject to a civil monetary penalty of not more than $ 10,000 for each act constituting such violation.

"(2) Procedure.—The provisions of section 1128A of the Social Security Act, other than subsections (a) and (b) and the first sentence of subsection (c)(1), shall apply to civil money penalties under this subsection in the same manner as such provisions apply to a penalty or proceeding under section 1128A of the Social Security Act.

"(3) Relation to hipaa.—Penalties shall not be imposed both under this subsection and under the regulations issued pursuant to section 264(c)(1) of the Health Insurance Portability and Accountability Act of 1996 (42 U.S.C. 1320d-2 note) for a single act or omission.

"(4) Equitable relief.—

"(A) In general.—Without limiting remedies available to other parties, a civil action may be brought by any aggrieved individual to enjoin any act or practice that violates subsection (e) and to obtain other appropriate equitable relief (including reinstatement, back pay, and restoration of benefits) to redress such violation.

"(B) Against state employees.—An entity that is a State or an agency of a State government may not assert the privilege described in subsection (a) unless before the time of the assertion, the entity or, in the case of and with respect to an agency, the State has consented to be subject to an action described in subparagraph (A), and that consent has remained in effect.

"(g) Rule of Construction.—Nothing in this section shall be construed—

"(1) to limit the application of other Federal, State, or local laws that provide greater privilege or confidentiality protections than the privilege and confidentiality protections provided for in this section;

"(2) to limit, alter, or affect the requirements of Federal, State, or local law pertaining to information that is not privileged or confidential under this section;

"(3) except as provided in subsection (i), to alter or affect the implementation of any provision of the HIPAA confidentiality regulations or section 1176 of the Social Security Act (or regulations promulgated under such section);

"(4) to limit the authority of any provider, patient safety organization, or other entity to enter into a contract requiring greater confidentiality or delegating authority to make a disclosure or use in accordance with this section;

"(5) as preempting or otherwise affecting any State law requiring a provider to report information that is not patient safety work product; or

"(6) to limit, alter, or affect any requirement for reporting to the Food and Drug Administration information regarding the safety of a product or activity regulated by the Food and Drug Administration.

"(h) Clarification.—Nothing in this part prohibits any person from conducting additional analysis for any purpose regardless of whether such additional analysis involves issues identical to or similar to those for which information was reported to or assessed by a patient safety organization or a patient safety evaluation system.

"(i) Clarification of application of hipaa confidentiality regulations to patient safety organizations.—For purposes of applying the HIPAA confidentiality regulations—

"(1) patient safety organizations shall be treated as business associates; and

"(2) patient safety activities of such organizations in relation to a provider are deemed to be health care operations (as defined in such regulations) of the provider.

"(j) Reports on Strategies to Improve Patient Safety.—

"(1) Draft report.—Not later than the date that is 18 months after any network of patient safety databases is operational, the Secretary, in consultation with the Director, shall prepare a draft report on effective strategies for reducing medical errors and increasing patient safety. The draft report shall include any measure determined appropriate by the Secretary to encourage the appropriate use of such strategies, including use in any federally funded programs. The Secretary shall make the draft report available for public comment and submit the draft report to the Institute of Medicine for review.

"(2) Final report.—Not later than 1 year after the date described in paragraph (1), the Secretary shall submit a final report to the Congress.

"Sec. 923. NETWORK OF PATIENT SAFETY DATABASES.

"(a) In General.—The Secretary shall facilitate the creation of, and maintain, a network of patient safety databases that provides an interactive evidence-based management resource for providers, patient safety organizations, and other entities. The network of databases shall have the capacity to accept, aggregate across the network, and analyze nonidentifiable patient safety work product voluntarily reported by patient safety organizations, providers, or other entities. The Secretary shall assess the feasibility of providing for a single point of access to the network for qualified researchers for information aggregated across the network and, if feasible, provide for implementation.

"(b) Data Standards.—The Secretary may determine common formats for the reporting to and among the network of patient safety databases maintained under subsection (a) of nonidentifiable patient safety work product, including necessary work product elements, common and consistent definitions, and a standardized computer interface for the processing of such work product. To the extent practicable, such standards shall be consistent with the administrative simplification provisions of part C of title XI of the Social Security Act.

"(c) Use of Information.—Information reported to and among the network of patient safety databases under subsection (a) shall be used to analyze national and regional statistics, including trends and patterns of health care errors. The information resulting from such analyses shall be made available to the public and included in the annual quality reports prepared under section 913(b)(2).

"Sec. 924. PATIENT SAFETY ORGANIZATION CERTIFICATION AND LISTING.

"(a) Certification.—

"(1) Initial certification.—An entity that seeks to be a patient safety organization shall submit an initial certification to the Secretary that the entity—

"(A) has policies and procedures in place to perform each of the patient safety activities described in section 921(5); and

"(B) upon being listed under subsection (d), will comply with the criteria described in subsection (b).

"(2) Subsequent certifications.—An entity that is a patient safety organization shall submit every 3 years after the date of its initial listing under subsection (d) a subsequent certification to the Secretary that the entity—

"(A) is performing each of the patient safety activities described in section 921(5); and

"(B) is complying with the criteria described in subsection (b).

"(b) Criteria.—

"(1) In general.—The following are criteria for the initial and subsequent certification of an entity as a patient safety organization:

"(A) The mission and primary activity of the entity are to conduct activities that are to improve patient safety and the quality of health care delivery.

"(B) The entity has appropriately qualified staff (whether directly or through contract), including licensed or certified medical professionals.

"(C) The entity, within each 24-month period that begins after the date of the initial listing under subsection (d), has bona fide contracts, each of a reasonable period of time, with more than 1 provider for the purpose of receiving and reviewing patient safety work product.

"(D) The entity is not, and is not a component of, a health insurance issuer (as defined in section 2791(b)(2)).

"(E) The entity shall fully disclose—

"(i) any financial, reporting, or contractual relationship between the entity and any provider that contracts with the entity; and "(ii) if applicable, the fact that the entity is not managed, controlled, and operated independently from any provider that contracts with the entity.

"(F) To the extent practical and appropriate, the entity collects patient safety work product from providers in a standardized manner that permits valid comparisons of similar cases among similar providers.

"(G) The utilization of patient safety work product for the purpose of providing direct feedback and assistance to providers to effectively minimize patient risk.

"(2) Additional criteria for component organizations.— If an entity that seeks to be a patient safety organization is a component of another organization, the following are additional criteria for the initial and subsequent certification of the entity as a patient safety organization:

"(A) The entity maintains patient safety work product separately from the rest of the organization, and establishes appropriate security measures to maintain the confidentiality of the patient safety work product.

"(B) The entity does not make an unauthorized disclosure under this part of patient safety work product to the rest of the organization in breach of confidentiality.

"(C) The mission of the entity does not create a conflict of interest with the rest of the organization.

"(c) Review of Certification.—

"(1) In general.—

"(A) Initial certification.—Upon the submission by an entity of an initial certification under subsection (a)(1), the Secretary shall determine if the certification meets the requirements of subparagraphs (A) and (B) of such subsection.

"(B) Subsequent certification.—Upon the submission by an entity of a subsequent certification under subsection (a)(2), the Secretary shall review the certification with respect to requirements of subparagraphs (A) and (B) of such subsection.

"(2) Notice of acceptance or non-acceptance.—If the Secretary determines that—

"(A) an entity's initial certification meets requirements referred to in paragraph (1)(A), the Secretary shall notify the entity of the acceptance of such certification; or

"(B) an entity's initial certification does not meet such requirements, the Secretary shall notify the entity that such certification is not accepted and the reasons therefor.

"(3) Disclosures regarding relationship to providers.— The Secretary shall consider any disclosures under subsection (b)(1)(E) by an entity and shall make public findings on whether the entity can fairly and accurately perform the patient safety activities of a patient safety organization. The Secretary shall take those findings into consideration in determining whether to accept the entity's initial certification and any subsequent certification submitted under subsection (a) and, based on those findings, may deny, condition, or revoke acceptance of the entity's certification.

"(d) Listing.—The Secretary shall compile and maintain a listing of entities with respect to which there is an acceptance of a certification pursuant to subsection (c) (2)(A) that has not been revoked under subsection (e) or voluntarily relinquished.

"(e) Revocation of Acceptance of Certification.—

"(1) In general.—If, after notice of deficiency, an opportunity for a hearing, and a reasonable opportunity for correction, the Secretary determines that a patient safety organization does not meet the certification requirements under subsection (a)(2), including subparagraphs (A) and (B) of such subsection, the Secretary shall revoke the Secretary's acceptance of the certification of such organization.

"(2) Supplying confirmation of notification to providers.—Within 15 days of a revocation under paragraph (1), a patient safety organization shall submit to the Secretary a confirmation that the organization has taken all reasonable actions to notify each provider whose patient safety work product is collected or analyzed by the organization of such revocation.

"(3) Publication of decision.—If the Secretary revokes the certification of an organization under paragraph (1), the Secretary shall—

    "(A) remove the organization from the listing maintained under subsection (d); and

    "(B) publish notice of the revocation in the Federal Register.

"(f) Status of Data After Removal from Listing.—

"(1) New data.—With respect to the privilege and confidentiality protections described in section 922, data submitted to an entity within 30 days after the entity is removed from the listing under subsection (e)(3)(A) shall have the same status as data submitted while the entity was still listed.

"(2) Protection to continue to apply.—If the privilege and confidentiality protections described in section 922 applied to patient safety work product while an entity was listed, or to data described in paragraph (1), such protections shall continue to apply to such work product or data after the entity is removed from the listing under subsection (e)(3)(A).

"(g) Disposition of Work Product and Data.—If the Secretary removes a patient safety organization from the listing as provided for in subsection (e)(3)(A), with respect to the patient safety work product or data described in subsection (f)(1) that the patient safety organization received from another entity, such former patient safety organization shall—

    "(1) with the approval of the other entity and a patient safety organization, transfer such work product or data to such patient safety organization;

"(2) return such work product or data to the entity that submitted the work product or data; or

"(3) if returning such work product or data to such entity is not practicable, destroy such work product or data.

"Sec. 925. TECHNICAL ASSISTANCE.

"The Secretary, acting through the Director, may provide technical assistance to patient safety organizations, including convening annual meetings for patient safety organizations to discuss methodology, communication, data collection, or privacy concerns.

"Sec. 926. SEVERABILITY.

"If any provision of this part is held to be unconstitutional, the remainder of this part shall not be affected."

(b) Authorization of Appropriations.—Section 937 of the Public Health Service Act (as redesignated by subsection (a)) is amended by adding at the end the following:

"(e) Patient Safety and Quality Improvement.—For the purpose of carrying out part C, there are authorized to be appropriated such sums as may be necessary for each of the fiscal years 2006 through 2010."

(c) GAO Study on Implementation.—

(1) Study.—The Comptroller General of the United States shall conduct a study on the effectiveness of part C of title IX of the Public Health Service Act (as added by subsection (a)) in accomplishing the purposes of such part.

(2) Report.—Not later than February 1, 2010, the Comptroller General shall submit a report on the study conducted under paragraph (1). Such report shall include such recommendations for changes in such part as the Comptroller General deems appropriate.

Speaker of the House of Representatives.

Vice President of the United States and President of the Senate.

Appendix B: American Nurses Association Position Statement on Medical Errors*

MEDICAL ERRORS

POSITION

ANA supports legislation that would mandate the reporting of medical errors to a National Center for Patient Safety. ANA maintains that this legislation must contain whistleblower protection to ensure that nurses who report medical errors are not retaliated against.

BACKGROUND

In 1999, the Institute of Medicine (IOM) issued a landmark report on patient safety, *To Err is Human: Building a Safer System*, which estimated that as many as 98,000 hospitalized patients die every year as a result of errors in their care. More Americans die annually from medical errors than from AIDS, automobile accidents, or breast cancer.

In 2003, the IOM released a companion to the medical errors report. This report, *Keeping Patients Safe: Transforming the Work Environment for Nurses*, recognized the critical role of nurses in patient safety, and recommended immediate reforms to the systems in which nurses work. These reforms include increasing the voice of staff nurses in hospital administration, increasing nursing staff, placing limits on the numbers of hours that a staff nurse may work (no more than 12 hours in a single shift and 60 hours in a 7 day period), and instituting a defined medical error and near miss reporting system that does not retaliate against reporters.

RATIONALE

ANA holds that errors in nursing care are rarely due to carelessness or incompetence, but rather that nurses work in complex systems that are prone to errors. ANA supports the development of a blame-free environment with open communication that enables workers to identify, study, and prevent medical errors.

The ANA contends that an over-reliance on individual scrutiny has failed to address the burgeoning system-wide problems that have fostered poor patient care. Patients must be assured that nurses and other health care professionals, acting within the scope of their expertise, will be able to speak for them without fear of retaliation.

Individuals who report medical errors must be able to do so in an environment that does not tolerate retribution. We must have a culture of awareness, not a culture of blame. Only when this happens will full reporting of medical errors be achieved.

CHAPTER 9

The Ethical Practice of the Psychiatric Advanced Practice Nurse in Public Mental Health Care

Barbara Jo Bockenhauer, RN, MSN, Kathleen Cummings, RN, and Lynette Hamlin, PhD, RN, CNM, FACNM

Learning Objectives

At the completion of this chapter, you will be able to:

1. Understand the ethical implications of the cultural evolution of public mental health care in the United States.
2. Recognize the challenges to ethical practice in public mental health care.
3. Discuss potential strategies to support autonomy of the individual with a serious and persistent mental illness.
4. Define informed consent in health care.
5. Discuss shared decision making between healthcare providers and patients.

John Ladd (1991) defined professional ethics as a "process of philosophical inquiry into the principles of morality of right and wrong conduct" (p. 130). Ethics are used to evaluate laws and customs but are not, in themselves, laws. Because ethics are grounded in culture, ethics change as the culture changes. With regard to the culture of mental illness, *plus que ca change, plus que reste la même chose,* or "The more it changes, the more it's the same thing."

How can the psychiatric advanced practice nurse provide care within a public mental health system that is ethically grounded in a culture that legislatively undermines autonomy as a core tenet of care? At what level can and should the advanced practice nurse intervene and in what capacity? Is coercive care a measure of advocacy and benevolence, or is it simply justice at the expense of the individual? Is the science of psychiatric mental health care supporting or undermining ethical practice?

This case presents the reality of "freeing" the individual with a serious and persistent mental illness from the restrictive institutions of care into what may be a no less restrictive freedom of our culture.

Part I: Clinical Example

Roger D. is in his mid-50s and appears to be in reasonable health, although he is unshaven and dressed in clothes that are dirty and disheveled. He reeks of urine and odors from the trash heap that was his bed and toilet for last night and for many prior nights. The vomitus on his jacket is several days old, and his pants zipper is broken. His pockets contain only slips of paper on which are written fragments of sentences, first names with partial phone numbers, and dollar amounts.

When the police arrive to investigate a report of suspicious behavior near a playground, Roger D. responds to their questioning with a string of expletives and raises his fists and charges at the police officers. He is sprayed with a toxic agent, handcuffed, and placed in the back of a squad car. After evaluating disposition options, one of the police officers delivers Roger D. to the community hospital for psychiatric evaluation. He is placed in an exam room and a hospital security officer is stationed outside the door.

Roger D. is seen by the psychiatric nurse practitioner for an evaluation. He is willing to participate in a discussion of his business plan and the injustice of his current state, but he is otherwise unwilling or unable to provide a history of his illness or contribute meaningfully to a plan for his care other than to say "Depakote is poisoning me." His clinical presentation does not indicate intoxication or gross head injury. However, Mr. D. refuses to have his blood drawn. His agitation and violent resistance to this intervention are managed by restraining his arms and legs with leather straps—"four-point restraints."

Roger D. remains restrained during the 5 hours it takes for the lab tests to confirm that he is not toxic from Depakote (divalproex sodium) and that his metabolic functions are within normal limits. Because Roger D. refuses the offer of voluntary psychiatric admission, the psych advanced practice nurse recommends involuntary commitment for a period of up to 10 days. Roger D. is transported, in handcuffs, to the designated receiving facility for involuntary psychiatric patients—the state hospital.

HISTORY, STIGMA, AND THE TRADITION OF COERCIVE TREATMENT OF THOSE WITH MENTAL ILLNESS

The surgeon general's report on mental health seeks to help reduce stigma by dispelling myths about mental illness, providing accurate knowledge to ensure more informed consumers, and encouraging help seeking by individuals experiencing mental health problems (Office of the Surgeon General, 1999). Although this is the first U.S. Surgeon General's report to address mental health problems, it is not the first time that an organized governmental approach to the issue of stigma and challenges of treating mental illness has been attempted.

A seventeenth-century culture grounded in Christian spirituality offered exorcism and efforts to "beat the devil" out of individuals displaying symptoms suggestive of a mental illness (Slovenko, 2003). The possessed who had no personal wealth were warehoused, chained, and beaten until their symptoms subsided or they were "released" through their own demise. Those with financial means had a more exclusive though no less restrictive option. In 1775, when Patrick Henry was demanding that he be given liberty or death, his own wife and mother of his six children was locked in the basement because she had "lost all her reason."

It was not until the end of the eighteenth century that the Frenchman Dr. Philippe Pinel and English Quakers led by William Tuke embraced moral treatment of individuals with mental illness—a perspective that offered a more humane, nonpunitive approach to care (Grob, 1992). In 1811, the Massachusetts Legislature established the Asylum for the Insane, now known as McLean Hospital, as one of the first U.S. facilities based on that principle. More important, this facility, and others like it, demonstrated that moral psychiatric treatment—sufficient food, kind words, and simple labor in a bucolic surrounding—could be effective. It was the potential for cure and restoration to productive social functioning that stimulated the development of state and private psychiatric hospitals as an alternative to jail for people with mental illnesses. A total of 18 of these facilities were in existence when Dorothea Lynde Dix began her crusade to reform conditions for mentally ill persons in jails and hospitals in the United States (Gruenberg & Archer, 1979). Care of people with mental illness in the United States, though continuing to be isolative, stopped being purposefully punitive.

The authority to direct an individual to the isolation of a psychiatric facility, without the individual's consent, is based on the sixteenth-century English *parens patriae* ruling (Slovenko, 2003). The king was recognized as the "father of the people," with the responsibility to act for those who were *non compos mentis*—insane. This legal precept was uniformly applied to ensure that the state could provide for the humane care of those individuals whose condition made it difficult, if not impossible, for them to care for themselves—a somewhat distorted application of the principle of beneficence. Routine harm and abuse were unfortunate and unplanned results of later economic forces.

Individuals committed to the asylum were disenfranchised from any source of power and without voting privileges in the same manner as women and African Americans of that era were. Many states had laws that provided that commitment could occur at the request of a husband, with the approval of the hospital. The introduction of a formal court process as part of commitment to the asylum was not instituted until late in the nineteenth century, as a result of one such wife's vigorous legal defense by her son. A role for a nurse educated to practice specifically with individuals who were mentally ill would not exist for almost the next 100 years.

Prior to the mid-1960s, the gentleman in this clinical example may have been committed to treatment for an indefinite period of time and required to take any medication ordered for the duration of his hospital stay (Gruenberg & Archer, 1979). His release from inpatient treatment would have been contingent on his willingness to continue treatment as an outpatient. It was not until the civil rights movement spawned a parallel mental health rights movement with similar goals, but arguably less successful outcomes, that respect for the rights of the individual with a mental illness would be championed.

The advanced practice nurse (APN) may make a recommendation that Roger D. be hospitalized, involuntarily, to protect the public and himself. In New Hampshire, the individual committed to a psychiatric hospital must have demonstrated behavior dangerous to self or others within the last 40 days or must demonstrate an inability to care for personal needs as a result of a mental illness (New Hampshire General Court, n.d.; New Hampshire Revised Statutes Annotated, 1986a). The statute specifically precludes its use in the case that an individual meets the criteria *only* because of the influence of alcohol or drugs or developmental delay. The APN's protection from liability for false imprisonment under these circumstances is incorporated into commitment law.

In addition to the right to due process, the involuntarily hospitalized psychiatric patient has both a right to treatment and a right to refuse treatment. More recently, the Americans with Disability Act has been referenced to support the right to receive treatment in the least restrictive environment. It is of concern to note that no consideration is given to whether the least restrictive environment can actually provide the appropriate treatment.

DISCUSSION QUESTIONS

1. Is there evidence of support of Roger D.'s autonomy in the process of his evaluation and commitment to involuntary hospitalization?
2. Is there a corollary authority of the state to involuntarily hospitalize the individual with unmanaged diabetes whose hyperglycemic state impairs his judgment behind the wheel?
3. What about the alcoholic individual?
4. Is the stigma of mental illness diminished or fueled by alternative, separate institutions for the care of individuals with a primarily mental health concern?

Part II: Involuntary Admission

The APN's recommendation to hospitalize Roger D. is supported by the authorizing physician, and Roger D. is transported, via sheriff's vehicle, to the state hospital. The admission process is similar to that which may occur in a general acute care hospital, with the notable exception that the patient is in shackles and has not asked for, nor agreed to, care. After gaining Roger D.'s commitment to act safely, the nurse directs that the shackles be removed and attempts to elicit the data needed to complete a full assessment. The patient offers long, rambling, tangential commentary in response to the questions being asked, though he specifically denies any psychiatric symptoms. He does admit to pain associated with the handcuffs, for which he requests "something strong." He accepts an offer of a sandwich but refuses to shower and permit an evaluation of his skin condition.

The nurse is concerned that sleeping on the streets has exposed Roger to infestation, assaults, and subsequent injury that may not have been addressed in the emergency department (ED). Because Roger demonstrated no gross evidence of physical impairment, the ED clinician listened to Roger's heart and lungs through his shirt. No evidence of his skin condition was provided in the ED assessment data. The inpatient psychiatric nurse considered whether this potential is of serious enough concern to institute a "personal safety emergency" in order to use physical force or the threat of force to effect the shower.

COERCIVE TREATMENT

A judge might find at the initial hearing (occurring within 72 hours of involuntary admission) that Roger D. should be held for evaluation for up to 10 days. The law that authorizes involuntary psychiatric hospitalization does not authorize involuntary treatment as part of that hospitalization (New Hampshire Revised Statutes Annotated, 1986b). Roger's right to treatment is protected under case law as well as state law, as is his right to refuse treatment. This includes the right to refuse medications as well as counseling, whether individually or in a group, and certainly a shower. Only if Roger D. demonstrates an "imminent risk" of harm to self or others can a further legal process be instituted to provide an essential treatment designed to resolve the emergency situation for a period up to 24 hours (De Nesnera & Folks, 2011). Should the imminent risk resolve within an hour, the emergency is considered resolved and no additional involuntarily administered treatments can be administered until and unless the patient's behavior again meets the imminent risk standard. The statute addressing this circumstance specifically precludes the administration of a long-acting or "depot" version of a medication as a treatment. An individual who has a serious mental illness and who is a danger to others may, though hospitalized, refuse any treatment likely to reduce the symptoms of illness. It is in this climate that the twenty-first-century psychiatric APN practices—classically described as one in which mental health patients are able to "die with their rights on."

DISCUSSION QUESTIONS

1. Under what, if any, circumstances does the nurse have a competing ethical responsibility that would justify infringing on Mr. D.'s right to refuse medication?

2. How is the principle of justice served when scarce healthcare resources are expended on those who refuse services?

Part III: Medication Administration

Roger D. contends that one particular clinician, a male mental health worker, can be trusted and agrees to have his shower supervised by that staff member. The mental health worker reports that Roger has some yellowing bruises on his shoulder and some red abrasions on his back, but no lacerations or rash-like skin conditions. After offering Roger D. another sandwich, which he accepts, the inpatient nurse begins a discussion about how best he can be helped. The topic of medication is addressed, and Roger D. suggests that he will take lithium carbonate "because it is natural" and a "vitamin."

INFORMED CONSENT AND ASSENT

The presumption of incompetence to consent to treatment is not a by-product of involuntary hospitalization (New Hampshire Revised Statutes Annotated, 1986b). Absent a judicial finding otherwise, individuals whose cognitive function may inhibit reasoning and insight *still* retain the capacity to give informed consent. However, the capacity to achieve full comprehension is not easily assessed through stated, or even written, declarations of understanding from the patient. In a psychiatric population, there is an even greater likelihood of assumption of inability to comprehend.

DISCUSSION QUESTIONS

1. How might the nurse use the therapeutic relationship in support of Roger D.'s decision to take the prescribed lithium?
2. Is the nurse meeting the ethical responsibility to provide informed consent if Roger D. agrees to take the lithium because he believes it is a vitamin?
3. Under what, if any, circumstances would it be ethical to withhold information in support of Roger D. agreeing to take a medicine?
4. By establishing an additional degree of oversight in conducting research with individuals who have a mental illness, is the Office of Human Subjects Protection supporting or undermining autonomy? Acting with beneficence? Ensuring justice?

The Office for Human Subjects Research Protection recognizes the status of individuals with a mental illness as members of a vulnerable population, requiring special accommodations to ensure that informed consent is legitimate (U.S. Department of Health and Human Services, 2009).

The guidelines for safe prescriptive practice include, but are not limited to, providing the information and guidance that will permit the patient to decide whether to take the medication—informed consent (American Nurses Association, 2007).

Part IV: Decision Making

The local mental health center faxes over the advance directives for psychiatric care that Roger D. had completed when he was stable. In them, he explains that lithium helps him become stable enough to consider restarting his Depakote, which is the medication that he prefers to take as a long-term intervention.

SHARED DECISION MAKING

Shared decision making is a partnership and interactive process between two experts—the client and the clinician—each sharing information and determining, collaboratively, the optimal treatment (Deegan & Drake, 2006). Patients are the experts on their own treatment preferences, values, and treatment goals. Clinicians have current, evidence-based practice information regarding diagnosis, course of illness, and treatment options. The essence of shared decision making is the expert clinician actively collaborating with the expert patient, with shared responsibility for the medical outcome (Adams & Drake, 2006).

The tradition of medical decision making is based on professional paternalism: The clinician prescribes a course of treatment that is followed by the patient. When the patient fails to follow the treatment as prescribed, the term *noncompliant* is applied. The reason for this noncompliance may be minimized or not even explored by the treating clinician.

Practicing within a shared decision-making model of care is a novel, and somewhat controversial, process for both patient and clinician. Some patients may want the physician to make all the decisions and will choose to participate in their treatment in a passive fashion. Other patients demand a more active role in the decision-making process. It is the responsibility of the APN to assess the patient preference in relation to shared decision making and to honor those preferences whenever possible.

Psychiatric APNs have the added responsibility of negotiating on behalf of the state's responsibility to protect (police power) and *parens patriae* (acting as parent). The psychiatric patient's ability to participate in shared decision making may be undermined by symptoms of impaired judgment and insight, as well as apathy. However, some mental health communities of clinicians have embraced the concept through the use of approaches described as client-centered care or negotiated decision making. Both terms refer to an approach that is grounded in excellent communication skills and engagement with the patient. Research supports that the more engaging the clinician's communication skills are, the greater the association with higher satisfaction, treatment adherence, and more successful outcomes for the mental health patient (Adams & Drake, 2006).

A nursing model provided by Ida Orlando (1961) captures the collaborative ideal described in shared decision making. Orlando notes that the nurse uses shared communication in determining the meaning of the patient's behavior, assessing the help required, and evaluating whether the patient was helped by the nurse's action. The Orlando communication model is well designed to support the APN's role in shared clinical decision making. The nurse uses the five senses to gather data about the patient, that is, see, smell, hear, taste, and touch. These data are then interpreted by the nurse into thoughts and feelings about the meaning of the behavior. The nurse then shares the thoughts and feelings about the behavior with the patient, thereby validating the meaning of the behavior. The APN can use this validation process to further the communication to incorporate the patient's desires with evidence-based practice.

There is a dearth of research in support of the shared decision-making process in relation to mental health. What little has been published supports that patients with mental illness benefit from the shared decision-making model. Mary Ellen Copeland provides leadership on this topic from the perspective of the psychiatric consumer. Her work with the Wellness, Recovery, Action Plan (WRAP) is being actively embraced by clinicians and patients (Copeland, 2011). She states:

> WRAP is a structured system to monitor uncomfortable and distressing symptoms that can help reduce, modify or eliminate those symptoms by using planned responses. This includes plans for how the patient wants others to respond when symptoms have made it impossible for you to continue to make decisions, take care of yourself, or keep safe. (p. 3)

DISCUSSION QUESTIONS

1. What are the parameters within which the APN can responsibly collaborate with involuntarily hospitalized patients in four-point restraints?
2. Are there legislative activities that would support or undermine the success of shared decision making with the psychiatric patient?

Part V: Homelessness and Mental Illness

Roger D. was a successful business owner in his community. His impulsive and irrational decision making, a product of his untreated bipolar disorder, led to the loss of his business. His irritability and hostility has cost him many close relationships, including his marriage and his ties with his children. Following his divorce, Roger repeatedly lost his alternative housing options because of his intimidating behavior in apartment houses, rooming houses, and shelters. With his own resources exhausted, Roger has been sleeping in an alley and eating from trashcans for the past few weeks. He will not apply for any assistance because he is in denial of the extent of his illness. He still believes that he is in the process of making a major business deal with the investors whose first names and partial phone numbers are on those slips of paper in his pocket. He is unaware of the irony that he is homeless and mentally ill in the community in which he grew up, owned a business, and staunchly resisted the inclusion of resources for those with mental illness—NIMBY (not in my backyard).

HOMELESSNESS

According to the Substance Abuse and Mental Health Services Administration (2011a), up to 407,000 people are homeless on any given night. Of this number, 26.2%, or approximately 107,000 people, have a serious mental illness. Approximately 34.7% of the homeless had chronic substance use issues (Substance Abuse and Mental Health Services Administration [SAMHSA], 2011a). The APN is challenged to provide psychiatric care as well as assistance in how to access food, shelter, and medical care and navigate the legal system. Nelson, Clarke, Febbraro, and Hatzipantelis (2005) noted, in a narrative study, that residents in supportive housing reported major improvements in their quality of life and a reduced rate of rehospitalization after the acquisition of a stable living situation. Residents also reported positive personal changes and increased independence and believed they had better access to resources such as food and clothing. Inadequate resources are the chronic challenge to managing the homeless situation among those with mental illness. Although the cost of maintaining a mentally ill patient in the hospital is greater than the price of the supported housing, there is little government assistance for this initiative. A homeless person with a mental illness may not qualify for Medicaid and will then be unable to defray the cost of appointments and medication.

In a study of 12 different communities across the country, general medical, mental health care, and state and local officials agreed that residential services were in short supply (Cunningham, McKenzie, & Taylor, 2006). These services included independent housing, group housing, transitional shelter, and supportive services. Subsidized housing vouchers are useless if there are no units to rent or the units are in communities that are resistive to supportive housing initiatives. Lack of housing lengthens hospital stays and may exacerbate symptoms that require rehospitalization. The absence of comprehensive and integrative mental health and substance abuse services presents the greatest challenge to stable placement of dually diagnosed patients.

Approximately 30% of people who are chronically homeless have mental health conditions, and approximately 50%

have co-occurring substance use problems (SAMHSA, 2011a). Because their symptoms may be active and often are untreated, these individuals have a difficult time negotiating basic needs for food, shelter, and safety. Their behavior causes distress to those who observe them. Their decision to avoid services is as likely to be based on their dissatisfaction with the circumstance of being involuntarily exposed to services or dissatisfaction with the services themselves—medications that cause unwanted effects. Creative strategies to support reengagement with these individuals include mobile outreach to provide convenient access to basic services, psychiatric treatment, and housing information as well as neighborhood-based drop-in centers.

Many people who are mentally ill and homeless end up in the criminal justice system (Cunningham, McKenzie, & Taylor, 2006; Slovenko, 2003). Slovenko referenced the term "transinstitutionalization" to describe the process by which mentally ill individuals are alternately (and often capriciously) remanded to either psychiatric or criminal justice systems. The evidence is suspect because definitions of mental illness are not standardized, but correctional facilities report a population in which 70% of all inmates have a mental illness. Thus, even with fewer involuntary psychiatric beds, the culture has identified a way in which those mentally ill individuals who need constant supervision receive it as a result of convictions for nonviolent crimes. Following release, these psychiatrically ill ex-convicts have limited eligibility for subsidized housing programs.

A weakness in the research related to the homeless mentally ill is that it is based on data obtained from shelters. The data do not account for the homeless who do not seek shelters or are utilizing nonconventional shelters. Mentally ill patients may choose homelessness for many reasons, including impaired judgment, exacerbation of symptoms, finances, or simply personal preference (Amador, 2007). There are no data to suggest that homeless mentally ill people choose incarceration; this is clearly the choice of the society in which the homeless mentally ill persons reside.

DISCUSSION QUESTIONS

1. Is it a choice for mentally ill individuals to remain homeless and at risk or a culturally imposed necessity?

2. If a choice, how does the nurse balance the autonomy and nonmaleficence principles?

3. If not a choice, what are the ethical implications of further nursing activism on local, state, and federal levels?

     The goals delineated by the 1999 Surgeon General's report reflect the values and beliefs of the current culture, while acknowledging the profound challenge in applying these culturally grounded standards to providing care for those with a mental illness. Ethical practice in the achievement of these goals can be elusive. Our culture demands that the individual seeking care assume responsibility for evaluating care options, using the healthcare professional as a consultant rather than decision maker. The clinician recommends care based on action-guiding theories of beneficence and nonmaleficence as well as autonomy and justice. It is, however, the case that individuals with a psychiatric illness often have a pronounced deficit in neurocognitive functioning that impedes judgment, insight, and motivation—the ability to exercise autonomy in a manner that leads to decisions that are good, not harmful, and respectful of the resources of the community. It is one of the fundamental paradoxes of mental health care—how to destigmatize an illness process that, even without an "asylum," isolates the individual from the culture to achieve these goals.

     With the coverage expansions under the Affordable Care Act and the Mental Health Parity and Addiction Equality Act, the goal is to provide broader coverage and access to traditional behavioral health care, but many recovery supports are not covered within our traditional medical framework (SAMHSA, 2011b). Advocates for mentally ill persons must work to ensure that access to behavioral health is included in all aspects of healthcare reform.

DISCUSSION QUESTION

1. How does the nurse support autonomy in the presence of impaired insight and judgment?

References

Adams, J. R., & Drake, R. E. (2006). Shared decision-making and evidence-based practice. *Community Mental Health Journal, 42*(1), 87–105.

Amador, X. (2007). *I am not sick I don't need help: How to help someone with mental illness accept treatment.* Peconic, NY: Vida Press.

American Nurses Association. (2007). *Psychiatric-mental health nursing: Scope and standards of practice.* Washington DC: Author.

Copeland, M. E. (2011). *Wellness recovery action plan.* San Francisco, CA: Peach Press.

Cunningham, P., McKenzie, K., & Taylor, E. F. (2006). The struggle to provide community-based care to low-income people with serious mental illnesses. *Health Affairs, 25*(3), 694–705.

Deegan, P. E., & Drake, R. I. (2006). Shared decision-making and medication management in the recovery process. *Psychiatric Services, 57*(11), 1636–1639.

De Nesnera, A., & Folks, D. G. (2011, Spring). Involuntary treatment for involuntary patients—evolution of the HE-M 306 rule in New Hampshire. *New Hampshire Bar Journal,* 58–61.

Grob, G. N. (1992). Mental health policy in America: Myths and realities. *Health Affairs, 11*(3), 7–22.

Gruenberg, E. M., & Archer, J. (1979). Abandonment of responsibility for the seriously mentally ill. *Milbank Fund Quarterly. Health and Society, 57*(4), 485–506.

Ladd, J. (1991). The quest for a code of professional ethics: An intellectual and moral confusion. In D. G. Johnson (Ed.), *Ethical issues in engineering* (pp. 130–136). Englewood Cliffs, NJ: Prentice Hall.

Nelson, G., Clarke, J., Febbraro, A., & Hatzipantelis, M. (2005). A narrative approach to the evaluation of supportive housing: Stories of homeless people who have experienced serious mental illness. *Psychiatric Rehabilitation Journal, 29*(2), 98–104.

New Hampshire General Court. (n.d.). Title X Public Health Chapter 135-C. New Hampshire Mental Health Services System. Nonemergency Involuntary Admissions. Section 135-C:45. Retrieved from http://www.gencourt.state.nh.us/rsa/html/X/135-C/135-C-45.htm

New Hampshire Revised Statutes Annotated. (1986a). 135-C:27 Involuntary emergency admission; criteria. Retrieved from http://nhrsa.org/law/135-c-27-involuntary-emergency-admission-criteria/

New Hampshire Revised Statutes Annotated. (1986b). 135-C:57 Treatment rights; rules. Retrieved from http://nhrsa.org/law/135-c-57-treatment-rights-rules/

Office of the Surgeon General. (1999). *Mental health: A report of the surgeon general.* Rockville, MD: National Institute of Mental Health.

Orlando, I. (1961). *The dynamic nurse–patient relationship: Function, process and principles.* New York, NY: Putman's Sons.

Slovenko, R. (2003). The transinstitutionalization of the mentally ill. *Ohio North University Law Review, 29*(3), 641–660.

Substance Abuse and Mental Health Services Administration. (2011a). Current statistics on the prevalence and characteristics of people experiencing homelessness in the United States. Rockville, MD: Author.

Substance Abuse and Mental Health Services Administration. (2011b). Leading change: A plan for SAMHSA's roles and actions 2011–2014 executive summary and introduction (HHS Publication No. [SMA] 11-4629 Summary). Rockville, MD: Author.

U.S. Department of Health and Human Services. (2009). *Code of Federal Regulations. Title 45 Public Welfare. Department of Health and Human Services. Part 46 Protection Of Human Subjects.* Retrieved from http://www.hhs.gov/ohrp/human-subjects/guidance/45cfr46.html

© Leksustiss/ShutterStock, Inc.

CHAPTER **10**

Healthcare Informatics

Robin Raiford, RN-BC, CPHIMS, FHIMSS, and Kathleen Kimmel, RN, BSN, MHA/MBA CPHIMS, FHIMSS

Learning Objectives

At the completion of this chapter, you will be able to:

1. Identify the five broad areas of informatics and healthcare technologies.
2. Discuss why it is important for all master's-prepared nurses to have knowledge and skills in these areas.
3. Critique the benefits and limitations of information technology related to patient care outcomes.
4. Evaluate tactics that incorporate ethical and legal protections in healthcare informatics.

Today's Informatics Landscape and Where We Are Headed

According to the World Health Organization, the United States spent more on health care per capita ($7,146) and more on health care as a percentage of its gross domestic product at 17.9% than any other nation in 2012 (World Health Organization, 2014), and that percentage grows every year. **Figure 10-1** comes from

215

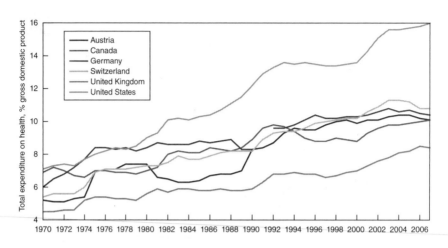

FIGURE 10-1 Healthcare cost rise, 1970–2007.

Source: Data from OECD Health Data, 2009.

the Organisation for Economic Co-operation and Development (OECD, 2009). U.S. healthcare costs are literally going off the chart and are well above the costs of the other five countries. Although it might be next to impossible for any healthcare professional to work harder in today's healthcare delivery system, everyone is going to need to work smarter and more efficiently in the future. These numbers support a belief held by an increasing proportion that the United States will not achieve high-value health care unless there is a broader system of linked goals and improvement initiatives. When Donald Berwick, a medical doctor, was named the administrator of the Centers for Medicare and Medicaid Services (CMS), he kicked off the "Triple Aim" initiative of improving the individual experience of care, improving the health of populations, and reducing the per capita costs of care for populations—in short, better health care, better health, at reduced costs (Berwick, Nolan, & Whittington, 2008).

Nurse managers are subject to pressure from The Joint Commission Core Measures, the Leapfrog Group, National Quality Forum, and Pay-for-Performance (P4P), to name a few. All of these initiatives are centered on ways to improve price and quality transparency in the current healthcare delivery model. Then, as if that were not enough, new delivery models are emerging to include patient-centered medical homes, patient-centered medical neighborhoods, and retail clinics, as well as employer-owned clinics. Change that focuses on how to get more out of the healthcare dollar is all around us.

Given all that is changing, nurse managers and informatics professionals can apply computer-assisted technology, which is referred to as informatics, as they address organizational work-flow productivity and operational efficiency or focus on disease and population management. Whether clinical informatics professionals' goals are saving money or saving patient lives or protecting quality of life of the population, they can apply technology to contribute to the success of these initiatives. Often, informatics professionals focus on all these goals.

Five broad areas of informatics are emerging, and they have a significant impact on today's healthcare market:

1. Executing strategic intent in the era of value-based care
2. Embracing the impact of meaningful use of electronic healthcare records
3. Developing secure external collaboration and patient engagement
4. Building clinically integrated networks
5. Designing business intelligence frameworks

Let's take a closer look at the high-level footprint of each of the five emerging informatics healthcare technologies areas.

EXECUTING STRATEGIC INTENT IN THE ERA OF VALUE-BASED CARE

The evolving incentives and payment models created by the U.S. Department of Health and Human Services force healthcare executives, including senior nurse executives, to think differently. We are moving from a "head 'em in—move 'em out" mentality in a fee-for-service volume-based care model into an environment where all caregivers need to work toward higher quality outcomes and accountability for all care given to a consumer. This includes taking care of consumers using preventive medicine and encouraging lifestyle habit changes while continuing to take care of consumers for short-term acute illness or chronic disease. This is not just about admission to discharge in a hospital, or check-in to check-out at the clinic; rather, it is about providing value-based care to Americans so that they can live healthy, productive lives as well as participate in their own health care. Shifting accountability to consumers for their well-being in a state of wellness, as well for resolution of acute care episodes, requires a large paradigm shift in thinking.

Value-based purchasing programs will be mandatory in a pay-for-performance program. The percentage of hospital inpatient payments will be withheld and then earned back based on quality performance and quality outcomes of the care. Also factored in will be the hospital's achievement of and improvement on selected clinical care, patient experience measures.

Additionally, in an effort to reduce the overall cost of care delivery, Medicare has created a voluntary program involving four bundled payment models. Models 1–3 provide retrospective reimbursement; models 2 and 3 include postepisode reconciliation; and model 4 offers single prospective payment. For all models, applicants must propose quality measures, which CMS will use to develop a set of standardized metrics. Last, Medicare began awarding Shared Savings contracts in 2012 to last a minimum of 3 years. Participating accountable care organizations (ACOs) must serve at least 5,000 Medicare beneficiaries, and their bonus potential will depend on Medicare cost savings plus the achievement of quality metrics. There is no escaping this trend. Healthcare practitioners must adapt to doing more with less and all the while working smarter. Literally, we need to get more "bang for the buck!"

Table 10-1 illustrates management strategies that need to be considered in this new era of greater risk as the country shifts to value-based care. Healthcare and nursing executives must shift the culture of their organizations to think about the patient "anytime, anywhere" and not just to think about what happens inside the walls of their organizations and within the confines of a "visit." In a global, high-level view, the length of stay is not a "visit"; rather, it is the length of someone's life. This means birth to death— not admission to discharge or check-in to checkout. What was once considered strategic in a fee-for-service world will change in an accountable care environment. Accountability, utilization, physician partnerships, technology investments, facility strategy, care coordination, and expense management take on entirely new meaning when we are forced to think outside the box and in terms of 24/7, what patients are doing 24 hours a day 365 days a year to manage their health and wellness. Patient engagement initiatives will explode the possibilities in the journey to transform health-care delivery.

TABLE 10-1 Management Strategies

Management Strategies	Fee for Service		Accountable Care
Accountability	Optimize performance within a single facility or organization	→	Optimize performance across all settings and time not dependent on a "visit"
Care coordination	Invest in only as an "avoidable losses" strategy	→	Develop high-performance partner network across healthcare spectrum of care
Expense management	Manage inpatient cost trend below revenue growth trend	→	Drive care to lowest-cost setting, which might be the phone or telemedicine
Facility strategy	Centralize and colocate acute care services	→	Widely distribute primary care, patient education, and preventive services
Physician partnerships	Align economically to drive acute care volumes higher	→	Align economically to manage shared risk
Technology investments	Win clinical technology "arms race," awards ("Most Wired")	→	Wire the health system for care coordination, interoperability, and collaboration
Utilization	Maximize acute care utilization	→	Redirect acute care to lower acuity settings, including telemedicine and patient-centered medical homes

EMBRACING THE IMPACT OF MEANINGFUL USE OF ELECTRONIC HEALTHCARE RECORDS

The impact of meaningful use of electronic healthcare records (EHRs) is leading the charge for redesigning basic care management and laying the foundation for the redesign of healthcare delivery. This is a multiyear initiative that has funding extending through 2021 (unless the statutory language in the American Recovery and Reinvestment Act [ARRA] is changed). Title XIII of ARRA, Health Information Technology, and Title IV of division B, may be cited as the "Health Information Technology for Economic and Clinical Health Act" or the "HITECH Act." However, it is most commonly referred to as "HITECH." HITECH put in place the statutory language for CMS to create the EHR incentive programs.

Make no mistake, the impact of the CMS EHR incentive programs, both for Medicare and Medicaid, is pushing this country forward in a way that was not achievable in the past 20 years. Meaningful use of an EHR means just that—use an EHR in a way that makes an impact, rather than the decades-old way of just tracking lab results and pharmacy orders. A challenge is that the EHR is often built on an antiquated information system infrastructure (i.e., legacy information systems), which were built in the 1970s or 1980s. Examples are billing and registration systems that decision makers are reluctant to change or upgrade because they perform their siloed functions well. Why change these systems when the registration and billing systems meet the immediate needs of the organization—to register patients and generate the bills?

CMS laid out three initial stages of meaningful use (MU) for the EHR incentive programs. During each of these stages, participants in the EHR incentive programs must achieve specified thresholds of defined functionality of the EHR in order to qualify to receive the incentive payment. Hence the term "meaningful use" was created. Without achieving MU thresholds, the incentive payment would not be distributed. The three initial stages are as follows:

Stage 1: Data Capture and Sharing. The initial stage focuses on increased implementation and adoption of EHR systems and capturing structured data, as well as beginning to use standardized vocabularies.

Stage 2: Advanced Clinical Processes. Stage 2 focuses on increased exchange of health information outside an organization's four walls, demonstrating care coordination across sites of care, and beginning to lay the foundation to empower patients with health information.

Stage 3: Improved Outcomes. The key focus of stage 3 is to build on the foundation of the two previous stages and drive the use of real-time data at the point of care, utilize outcomes-focused clinical quality measures, utilize clinical decision support for prevention, disease management, and safety as well as provide access to patient self-management tools.

All of this activity creates an opportunity for nursing managers and healthcare informatics professionals at a national level to tackle this new challenge head on and be successful. Think of the goal of having every acute care hospital in the United States effectively using EHRs as part of a plan to eventually connect the data.

In many ways the goal to create a clinical data "electronic highway" is akin to the building of the interstate highway system back in the Eisenhower administration. The need for an efficient and effective high-speed highway system was seen as essential for national security, allowing troops and supplies to move quickly between coasts and borders in the event of war. The Federal Aid Highway Act of 1956 created the legislative language for the national federal highway system we have today. In many ways, the HITECH Act's meaningful use incentive program is similar to the Highway Act because it lays the foundation for a new electronic highway that captures and shares patient data to achieve safer, higher-quality, more efficient care. CMS and the Office of the National Coordinator (ONC) are spearheading this effort to build a new toll road for healthcare delivery for the United States. CMS and ONC efforts are also supported by the National Institute for Standards and Technology, which oversees standards to be used in federal programs.

DEVELOPING SECURE EXTERNAL COLLABORATION AND PATIENT ENGAGEMENT

Now more than ever before, there is an emphasis on secure external collaboration and patient engagement. It is no longer acceptable to hoard relevant patient data within the four walls of the organization. To achieve stage 2 MU, organizations need to transmit summary of care records electronically for 10% of all discharges, submit immunization data in accordance with applicable law and practice, and develop standards to facilitate exchange using entity- and provider-level directories. Organizations will need to build consumer confidence that the patient portal and Internet-based communication is secure, as well as evaluate the role of personal health records (PHRs) and portals in patient engagement. Healthcare providers, both ambulatory and hospital based, will be responsible for driving patient use of tools.

BUILDING CLINICALLY INTEGRATED NETWORKS

A clinically integrated network would be an ideal IT environment. It would represent a common workflow—access to consistent applications across all modalities of care. Physician offices, hospitals, home health, postacute, and long-term care facilities would all feed data into an enterprise data warehouse or a variety of specific use data marts. Although that looks wonderful on a diagram, in reality, it does not exist in many locations around the country. Many wonder if we will see this ideal network widespread across the country in our lifetimes.

In an ideal world, the ACO would have a common enterprise architecture used throughout all modalities of care. But we know that this is not realistic in the vast majority of healthcare organizations today. In most cases, healthcare organizations have very little connectivity from the ambulatory clinics or hospital IT environments to the postacute care world. For example, most long-term postacute care (LTPAC) facilities have little if any clinical automation to support care delivery, and most have limited budgets to implement this functionality. Connecting the various care modalities and venues into the ACO will require new solutions and technologies. Continuing the highway analogy, acute care hospitals, which were eligible for funding, were able to pave their access to the electronic healthcare highway, but LTPAC facilities and specialty hospitals, such as rehabilitation and psychiatric facilities, were excluded by law from that particular funding opportunity. All healthcare delivery providers will need to be in the loop of care coordination to be successful in an ACO model.

DESIGNING BUSINESS INTELLIGENCE FRAMEWORKS

Building a business intelligence framework will be key to developing a thoughtful system of care out of the ad hoc processes in use today. Whether we like it or not, we are now entering an era of value-based care, shared savings plans, and bundled payments. Organizations cannot ignore the fact that it will be essential for nurse managers, advanced practice nurses, and health informatics professionals to understand the key concepts of business intelligence. This includes reviewing descriptive, prescriptive, and prescriptive analytic models to evaluate enhanced workflows, productivity, and patient care outcomes.

The Importance of Nurse Knowledge and Skills in the Five Areas of Informatics

Current IT systems are hampered by basic challenges and the symptoms of disparate, heterogeneous systems. Nurse managers and healthcare informatics professionals frequently hear comments such as, "I can't access my images at my office across town" and "My patient doesn't know whether she's allergic to this drug, and I can't tell from her records." Or they might hear the frequent complaint, "We've done the same test three times because there was no easy way of knowing" or "Our systems can't speak to each other." All the while, nurse managers and healthcare informatics professionals are asked to take action, to do something about this, and to tell the information systems department to just fix it, and fix it now. All of which is easier said than done. Changing workflow in an electronic healthcare record is a journey, not a destination, and it cannot happen overnight.

Nurse managers and healthcare informatics professionals will be increasingly expected to be informed and to use their knowledge to provide advice and direction during the decision-making process. Nurses are key stakeholders in a large, complex information system arena. This section begins a closer look at the nursing informatics role. Included is a discussion of the five broad areas of informatics and healthcare technologies and how the nurse informaticist can function in relation to these areas.

THE ROLE OF NURSING INFORMATICS IN STRATEGY EXECUTION IN THE ERA OF VALUE-BASED CARE

New incentives and greater risk characterize industry transformation. A paradigm shift in thinking is required. We cannot keep doing business the old way of the 1970s, when Dr. Kildare and Marcus Welby, MD, were the only doctors you ever saw in your community. As nurses, we need to realize that we lost out to wearing our nursing caps in the 1980s and that nursing will lead the charge to getting rid of paper in the twenty-first century. We need to stop charting like Florence Nightingale is the head nurse on 8 West!

It might be a stretch for the bachelor's-prepared nurse to realize the impact, but it is essential for master's- and doctorally prepared nurses to realize this shift in the domains of accountability, responsibility, and thinking. Regardless of whether your organization is an ACO, all organization are eventually going to need to function like an ACO to survive financially in the changing healthcare delivery landscape.

Management imperatives for nurse managers, as well as healthcare informaticists, will shift, moving from fee for service to an accountable care model. None of us can work harder in today's fast-paced world, but we all must work smarter, and that includes embracing information technology. Accountability will shift from optimizing performance within the facility to optimizing performance across care settings and across time. Utilization will go from maximizing acute care utilization to redirecting acute care to a lower acuity setting and decreasing readmission rates. Physician partnerships will change from aligning economically to drive acute care volumes to aligning economically to manage shared risk. Care coordination will go from a "nice to have" to a "must have." No longer will investing in an avoidable-losses strategy in a fee-for-service model help the organization survive. What is needed is a shift in thinking and actions to develop a high-performance partner network across the entire continuum of care, including long-term and postacute care settings.

On the information technology front, nursing leaders must help influence the need to move from winning a clinical technology "arms race" to how to wire the healthcare system for coordination and collaboration. This includes a shift in thinking toward interoperability and making health information exchange (HIE) a verb in your organization—not HIE the noun, such as the hospital across town that belongs to the local regional health information organization (RHIO). Facility strategies will need to be altered from centralized and colocated acute care services to widely distributed primary care and preventive services networks. Another area affected by the changing healthcare landscape is expense management because healthcare executives are forced to move from managing inpatient cost trends below the revenue growth trend to driving care to lowest-cost settings.

THE ROLE OF NURSING INFORMATICS IN A WORLD OF MEANINGFUL USE OF ELECTRONIC HEALTHCARE RECORDS

The nursing informatics role in the meaningful use arena sets the stage for redesigning basic care management. It lays a foundation for redesigning healthcare delivery with a heavy focus on standardized vocabulary, patient engagement, and coordination of care, including information exchange between providers of care. Depending on the size of the organization, several nurse informaticists might be assigned to achieving meaningful use. Their efforts involve evaluation of the exact objective and measure required to be achieved for meaningful use as well as following any standards and implementation guides that were defined in the regulation. Capturing the required data elements is essential to achieving accurate numerators for attestation purpose. In a very large organization, following the technical requirements to achieve meaningful use can absolutely be a full-time position.

While one informaticist might be focused on the EHR technical details in the configuration and build, another team led by another nurse manager or nurse informaticist will need to focus on the clinician process of capturing required data elements. This process might involve having physician and nurse champions of the EHR to establish momentum and lead the training needed to engage the staff in what might seem to be needless data entry. This pivotal change in behavior must be embraced by staff to ensure compliance with the data capture to achieve desired thresholds and ultimately to provide the foundation for improved patient outcomes.

THE ROLE OF NURSING INFORMATICS IN SECURE EXTERNAL COLLABORATION AND PATIENT ENGAGEMENT

Healthcare organizations will soon need to identify the stakeholders who have the authority and are responsible and accountable for making decisions to lay a solid foundation for patient engagement activities. These stakeholders could include a team consisting of representatives from nursing, marketing, and communications. Regardless of the stakeholder participants, it is the outcome that truly matters. Indeed, to achieve meaningful use an organization must ensure that 50% of patients have access to view, download, or transmit their healthcare data and that 5% of patients actively do view, download, or transmit their health information to a third party. This includes either a wide-scale patient portal or personal health record product to achieve these measures.

Nurse managers, as well as nurse informaticists, must engage in stakeholder discussions to determine the strategies to engage these patients. Will these strategies be applied to different types of patients, a certain patient population, or the entire patient population? Decisions need to be made regarding how to make patient engagement more visible (e.g., patient engagement campaign, patient focus groups, or consumer incentives) for both internal and external customers. The role of patients and families (e.g., patient advisory council) must be determined and a governance structure needs to be developed. The phrase "it takes a village" certainly applies to this new initiative to actively involve patients in disease management and overall health and wellness plans.

THE ROLE OF NURSING INFORMATICS IN BUILDING CLINICALLY INTEGRATED NETWORKS

Another significant challenge for most organizations is the ability to monitor patients in home care situations. The ability to collect medical device or monitor data and evaluate them against data acquired in other environments is a key success factor for using clinical decision support to improve quality of care while also eliminating avoidable costs or high-cost interventions that are not supported by evidence-based protocols of care. Care teams need to have the most current patient data available and must be able to update these data in real time to avoid medical errors and to provide and document the interventions taken to stabilize or improve the health status of patients. Failure to achieve a clinically integrated network will result in an inability to improve quality and cost efficiencies— for example, admissions or readmissions into more expensive care modalities.

In an ideal world, the ACO uses a common enterprise architecture for all modalities of care. But this is not realistic in the vast majority of healthcare organizations today, and it certainly presents a challenge for chief information officers and informatics professionals. In most cases healthcare organizations have very little connectivity to the postacute care world. In an age of MU of EHRs, we are just now defining more significant exchange of information. Nurse informaticists play a key role in incorporating LTPAC facilities and other venues of care with little or no clinical automation into supporting care delivery. Connecting the various care modalities and venues of care into the ACO requires new solutions and technologies.

THE ROLE OF NURSING INFORMATICS IN DESIGNING BUSINESS INTELLIGENCE FRAMEWORKS

A business intelligence framework within a healthcare organization is quickly becoming a must-have rather than a nice-to-have tool. Doing more with less—less human resource power, less revenue—means getting the most bang out of every single buck that flows through the organization.

Business intelligence is key to developing a thoughtful system of care from the ad hoc processes that we employ today. Organizations need to move from dashboards, reports, and graphs, or "what happened," to looking at what might happen or what should happen.

Informatics professionals will be required to rely on their knowledge of clinical workflow to review statistical models, forecasts, and simulations of what-if analyses. With these tools, they can answer questions regarding impact on patient outcomes, lengths of stay, and reimbursement. Predictive modeling is an extremely valuable tool for nurse managers in today's world of tight budgets and staffing challenges.

Finally, in organizations with advanced business intelligence frameworks, and advanced clinical processes for capturing data electronically, prescriptive analytics comes into play to answer the question, What should we do? The answer can be found by using mathematical models and linear programming to determine when to change equipment, medication source, or brands for supplies. This level of prescriptive analytics can have an impact on overall operating budget as well as patient outcomes. Although statisticians can be insightful in analysis of the numbers, nurse managers and nursing informaticists must interpret the overall impact on clinical operations, patient care, patient satisfaction, and patient outcomes, not just the impact on the bottom line of the budget.

The Benefits and Limitations of Information Technology Related to Patient Care Outcomes

The benefits of information technology affecting patient care outcomes today have been severely limited because of the lack of standardized vocabularies and standard formats for objects in EHRs. The endless possibilities for clinical decision support (CDS) are about to explode in this country because of the fact that MU of EHRs is forcing data to be captured using standardized vocabularies.

Nurse managers and healthcare informatics professionals will begin to see less emphasis on technology and more focus on a careful selection of change targets and sensitivity to clinical process. Is there a sustainable workflow in process, or is it hit or miss depending on what day it is and who is working? There is also a trend in greater emphasis on guidance-based CDS, less on interruptive mechanisms, and a growing appreciation of the importance of managing CDS appropriately. Prior to the introduction of EHRs, when nurses identified a need for a new workflow they created a new form to complete. In the world of EHRs, nurses must be cautious about managing an electronic workflow by creating a new rule. As rules proliferate and alerts and reminders multiply, "alert fatigue," which occurs when users are bombarded with alerts that consume the workflow, causes users to see alerts as noise or nuisances, such that they become numb to them. When this occurs, the alerts become meaningless. CDS systems need to have solid governance and clinical knowledge management built in to design to anticipate unintended consequences and track compliance with alerts. All in all, there is more pressure than ever to reduce costs and improve the quality of care in a measurable way.

The Agency for Healthcare Research and Quality (AHRQ, 2012) report, *Enabling Patient-Centered Care through Health Information Technology*, contains an extensive literature review of more than 327 articles on the benefits and barriers to information technology related to patient-centered care. This publication was based on research conducted by the Johns Hopkins University Evidence-based Practice Center (EPC). The study results suggested the positive effects, collectively cited in the more than 327 articles, of patient-centered care enabled by health IT interventions on healthcare process outcomes, disease-specific clinical outcomes, intermediate outcomes, responsiveness to the needs and preferences of patients, shared decision making, patient–clinician communication, and access to medical information. As organizations and legislators seek to gain validation that federal dollars allocated to this effort are achieving the intended results of improved patient safety and improved patient outcomes, MU of EHRs will continue to be a hot topic for the foreseeable future.

TACTICS THAT INCORPORATE ETHICAL AND LEGAL PROTECTIONS IN HEALTHCARE INFORMATICS

The very dynamic and fast-growing topic of ethical and legal protections in healthcare informatics is the subject matter of an increasing number of books in the United States and international markets. The World Wide Web, Twitter, and social media sites have an impact on health care and are creating challenges for incorporating ethical and legal protections in healthcare informatics. This presents the challenge of incorporating ethical and legal protections well beyond personal health records and patient portals.

At the first level, to incorporate ethical and legal protections into healthcare informatics and to protect personal health information, nurse managers and nurse informaticists must actively engage in security and privacy risk analysis. Perhaps for the first time in their professional lives, nurse managers and nurse informaticists will need to familiarize themselves with the rules in the Code of Federal Regulations (CFR) that pertain to the protection of health information. They must be aware of administrative as well as physical and technical safeguards relating to protecting personal health information.

CASE STUDY: *Executing Strategic Intent in the Era of Value-Based Care*

During a webinar on December 4, 2012, titled "Translating Meaningful Use into Meaningful Outcomes," the presenter, Rich Boehler, MD, president and chief executive officer of St. Joseph Healthcare, Nashua, New Hampshire, spoke of his experience as chief medical officer of St. Joseph Medical Center in Towson, Maryland (Boehler, 2012). There he used medical staff performance dashboards to dramatically improve outcomes and lower both costs and lengths of stay. Boehler began using clinical and business intelligence applications to address the wide variation in clinical care. In this case he chose to look at the differences between colorectal surgeons' and general surgeons' approaches to a common diagnosis-related group (DRG): Major Large and Small Bowel (DRGs 329 and 330). This involved surgical cases for both benign and malignant disease. In many organizations both general surgeons and colorectal surgeons manage these patients. Often one studies physician variation within the context of a single division. In this case, because both the colorectal surgeons and general surgeons performed major large and small bowel operations, both divisions were studied.

Boehler (2012) used analytics to study three surgical techniques, including robotic, open, and laparoscopic surgery. He used the analytics to show the wide variation between the general surgeons and the colorectal surgeons to start interdepartmental communication. The results were profound. In joint departmental meetings both types of surgeons discussed their techniques and the associated outcomes in a cooperative, collegial manner. Both types of surgeons, colorectal and general, were eager to learn and assist each other. The result of an analytics-based conversation was that all surgeons, whether they were colorectal or general surgeons, experienced a noticeable improvement in outcomes. That is, every surgeon improved. The patients were the true beneficiaries. The hospital achieved some noticeable financial gains. In aggregate, the combined clinical and financial outcomes equated to a length of stay reduction and a cost savings of $11,000 per case.

DISCUSSION QUESTIONS

1. In the case study, why were visual analytical applications (e.g., scorecards and dashboards) instrumental in changing the behavior of the surgeons?

2. Why is collecting, providing, and displaying data important when preparing to meet with clinicians?

3. In this case, when physicians were presented with analytical data on performance they began to collaborate and share best practices, and each physician improved. Is this a one-time scenario or can it be successfully duplicated across most clinical quality care situations and surgical and medical departments? Why or why not?

Embracing the Impact of Meaningful Use
of Electronic Healthcare Records

MU of EHRs is the cornerstone of the EHR Incentive Programs federal program, designed to encourage the adoption of health information technology (HIT) by physicians and hospitals. The program includes incentive payments for meeting defined criteria for the implementation and usage of advanced clinical information systems.

The old English saying "Mind your Ps and Qs" was said to schoolchildren to urge them to be careful and diligent with their penmanship. MU nurse managers also need to mind their Ps. That is, clinicians frequently lump MU project-related vernacular into one big bucket. Indeed, the four Ps need to be carefully distinguished:

- *Project:* The project includes issues, tasks, communication, planning, and escalation that relate to the project.
- *Process:* The process refers to the workflow. It includes the process of collecting the data: order entry, vital signs, prescriptions, discharge planning, and so forth.
- *Product: Product* refers to the features and functions of the EHR, including orders, results, electronic medication administration report (eMAR), clinical documentation, appointments, and so forth.
- *Portfolio: Portfolio* refers to a collection of projects that can affect a department or organization. Examples of projects that together create a portfolio can be an ACO, International Statistical Classification of Diseases and Related Health Problems (ICD-10), patient satisfaction, meaningful use, and physician quality reporting system (PQRS).

Not minding your Ps can create chaos and introduce risks for failure. One person cannot do this alone—it truly takes a village.

In working with MU or any other HIT-enabled project, it is helpful to distinguish between people, process, and technology. What's more, one needs to be cognizant of the portfolio of projects that are under way. Chances are your organization may be simultaneously working on multiple projects such as implementing an ACO, MU, PQRS, value-based purchasing (VBP) initiatives, and 30-day readmission monitoring, among others. Often the same resources need to be involved or assigned to these efforts. Your program office, which is also referred to as a project office, usually manages the status of projects, assigning each project a project manager to ensure that it is on track and within budget. Your program office, in conjunction with your executive leaders, is charged with prioritizing the various projects. Prioritization of the project backlog should be in alignment with your organization's strategic plan.

A common mistake is to assume that an investment in technology will solve anything and that process and infrastructure will naturally fall into place. Actually, technology is the first step. The much larger work effort is to use the technology, especially EHRs, in a clinical business intelligence capacity to derive analytics for performance management initiatives (**Figure 10-2**).

The project itself, with the corresponding issues, planning, monitoring, tracking, reporting, engaging of stakeholders, escalating, and so forth, is a major effort. The people part, which includes various stakeholders and users, is your largest effort (**Figure 10-3**). It dwarfs everything else. When discussing people, the concepts of buy-in, engagement, adoption, and culture come into play. Communication, both in formulating compelling

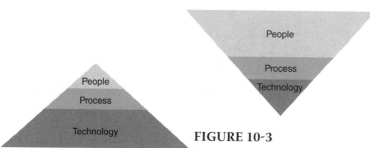

FIGURE 10-2
The perception is that technology is the biggest effort.

FIGURE 10-3
The reality is that communications and the people component of performance management are where the most effort must be expended.

messages that unite and are tied to your organization's core principles and values, is vital.

The people part of the equation requires communication through the three project phases (**Figure 10-4**):

1. *Preparation and planning phase:* The communications in this stage focus on contacting and creating what is being done and why.
2. *Acceptance phase:* The acceptance phase embraces the principles of change management. It focuses on understanding the change and uses communication to build a positive perception.
3. *Communication phase:* As implementation nears, the communication that has occurred in the prior phases builds to support adoption, institutionalization, and internalization. Inadequacies in communication in the previous two phases are a setup for failure or major obstacles to overcome. How do you know whether

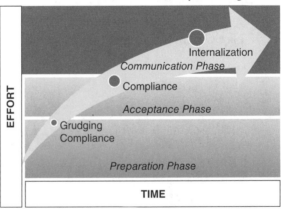

FIGURE 10-4   Success in all three phases is iterative and builds on itself to reach the internalization stage. If communication does not build commitment, a project can suffer from mediocre compliance and be at risk.

there has been inadequate communications? It is easy to tell because the language of the stakeholders and users often demonstrates grudging compliance such as, "It is just another thing they are forcing on us." Another failure or obstacle is formal versus genuine compliance. The difference is subtle. Formal compliance is flat acceptance, whereas genuine compliance indicates that stakeholders and users agree with the technology, the implementation, and how the technology is being used.

CASE STUDIES

CASE 1: MEANINGFUL USE

Tenet Healthcare Corporation, in Dallas, Texas, with 49 hospitals in 10 states, built an enterprise data warehouse to measure, monitor, and track (attest to) MU. Tenet's clinical business intelligence approach allowed 53% of its hospitals to attest as of October 2012. The MU program is monitored to track clinical improvements and waste reduction. A September 2012 Institute of Medicine report estimated that health care could cut the heavy financial burden by roughly a third, or nearly $765 billion every year, by reducing money wasted through the provision of unnecessary services, inefficiently delivered services, excessive prices, and burdensome administrative fees. In terms of eliminating waste, Tenet claims its MU program has accomplished the following:

- Decreased duplicate lab tests by 2.8%
- Trimmed duplicate radiology tests by 2.4%
- Reduced printing costs by more than $1 million

What's more, Tenet estimates MU has identified 2,381 potential adverse drug events and has decreased adverse medication administration events by 0.8%. Tenet, a for-profit hospital chain, estimates that starting in 2013, MU will have a positive financial impact on earnings before interest, taxes, depreciation, and amortization (Johnson & Browne, 2012).*

---

*No updates available at time of publication.

DISCUSSION QUESTIONS

1. Discuss nursing's role in the planning, acceptance, and communication phases of achieving MU.

2. Leadership in aligning people, processes, and technologies is an important best practice. In many ways it requires a collaborative community organizer skill set. Are nurses best suited for assuming a community organizer role within their organizations? Why or why not?

*****

CASE 2: DEVELOPING SECURE EXTERNAL COLLABORATION AND PATIENT ENGAGEMENT

During the January 30, 2013, Integrating the Healthcare Enterprise Connectathon Conference in Chicago, Jamie Ferguson, in his keynote address titled "Achieving the Vision of Safer and Higher Quality Care," reported that mobile application usage on various mobile devices is approaching a 50% usage rate. Kaiser patients access the web portal, request online e-refills, and use online appointment applications.

Ferguson (2013) discussed some impressive results that stem from health information technology–enabled patient engagement. For example, patients who are engaged collaboratively with their care team were noted to exhibit the following characteristics:

- Exceed the national high-risk patient cholesterol guidelines by 40%

- Experience a 24% lower probability of death from heart attack and a 62% lower probability of serious heart attacks

- Have a 90% lower mortality from second heart attacks

Ferguson also reported that high patient satisfaction appears to be correlated with high levels of HIT-enabled patient engagement, including the following:

- Higher patient involvement in care

- Increased use of scheduled e-visits—800% higher

- Increased use of secure messaging with physicians—more than 600%

Perhaps one of the most impressive statistics Ferguson quoted was that highly engaged HIT-enabled patients had 24% fewer office visits. At a time when this nation is striving to provide better care at lower costs, HIT-enabled patient engagement is showing great promise (Ferguson, 2013).

DISCUSSION QUESTIONS

1. Describe how nurses can promote technologies that engage patients in their care.

2. Discuss how to evaluate the effectiveness of technologies that engage patients in their care.

3. In the case study, Kaiser had high levels of patient engagement. What methods can nurses use to duplicate Kaiser's success and achieve higher levels of patient engagement?

*****

CASE 3: BUILDING CLINICALLY INTEGRATED NETWORKS

As the U.S. healthcare industry moves from fee-for-service reimbursements to value-based purchasing, attention often shifts overseas for examples from other countries. The National Health Service (NHS) in the United Kingdom has been continually working to enhance its clinically integrated networks (CINs). Clinical and business intelligence analytics are at the core of the NHS's efforts.

The Bexley Care Trust is part of the NHS South East London borough of Bexley. Bexley Care Trust launched an analytical CIN system. The system included a suite of locally adapted reporting solutions that provides meaningful data to help general practitioners make appropriate care decisions to manage referrals, monitor prescribing patterns, track spending by each physician, analyze vital signs data, and study adherence to quality indicators. Decisions are no longer haphazard; instead, decisions are supported by data. In addition, a distributive leadership model has emerged as a result of physicians working collaboratively with the patient. From April to December 2011, the number of hospital admissions declined by 289 from the number of admissions during the same period the previous year. The cost savings in the 6-month study period were £267,000.

DISCUSSION QUESTIONS

1. The Bexley Care Trust case study took place in the United Kingdom, which has a nationalized health system. Focusing on the universal challenge our two countries share of improving quality and lowering costs, how can this example be applied to the U.S. healthcare system?

2. In the United Kingdom, the Bexley Care Trust measures and monitors clinicians' care decisions such as referrals, prescribing patterns, costs of care, and adherence to quality standards. In the United States, as we shift from volume- to value-based accountable care, is it important to track these dimensions of care? Why or why not?

3. Are there any ethical considerations to tracking and monitoring physician/clinician care decisions? Are there other methods that can be used to reduce variability of care and ensure compliance with standards of care?

Executing Strategic Intent in the Era of Value-Based Care

The concept of value-based healthcare purchasing (VBP) is that providers of health care need to be held accountable for both cost and quality of care. VBP brings together information on the quality of health care, including patient outcomes and health status combined with data on costs. It focuses on managing the use of the healthcare system to reduce inappropriate care, locate and reduce waste, and identify and reward the best-performing providers. At the very core of VBP are clinical surveillance practices. Clinical surveillance uses advanced statistical predictive modeling techniques that incorporate historical data from chronic disease patients and simulate the types of care and treatments that are most likely to result in a positive outcome. As nurses collect and enter data in EHRs, they contribute to the capture of data that can be analyzed to guide clinicians in the care of populations of patients.

CASE STUDY: *Practice Guidelines for Better Care*

Jonathan B. Perlin, MD, PhD, president of Clinical and Physicians Services Group, and chief medical officer at the Hospital Corporation of America, was a panelist at the February 4, 2013, *Health Affairs* briefing. He described some examples of better care. He provided an example from Kaiser Permanente. In 2008, Kaiser reported on its Healthy Bones Program, which developed measures to proactively identify patients who are high risk for developing osteoporosis and hip fractures. Using practice guidelines, home health, and education resulted in a 37% reduction in hip fractures and as high as a 50% reduction among those at risk.

DISCUSSION QUESTIONS

1. Identifying at-risk patients with predictive analytical models is one thing; gaining patient engagement and ownership of their medical conditions is another. Discuss how the role of the nurse in patient education could increase patient compliance.

2. Clinical surveillance involves predictive analytics aimed at identifying at-risk populations and proactively intervening. What is the nurse's role in proactively identifying at-risk patients?

Designing Business Intelligence Frameworks

Nurse managers have a lot of latitude in designing business intelligence frameworks. Nurse managers and nursing informatics professionals should consider selecting a process used by their organization. Popular options are the Plan-Do-Study-Act cycle that is recommended by the Institute for Healthcare Improvement. Other popular quality improvement processes are Lean and Six Sigma. (Some organizations combine Lean and Six Sigma into one process called Lean Six Sigma.) Business intelligence uses electronic data. Chances are the data in the organization's EHRs can be used to provide the data on which to make decisions. These data are rolled into the quality improvement process to drive the performance management initiatives that need to occur to improve outcomes.

CASE STUDY: *Framework Design*

An example of a framework design was published in the February 2013 issue of *Health Affairs*. In the article "HealthPartners' Online Clinic for Simple Conditions Delivers Savings," Courneya, Palattao, and Gallagher (2013) of HealthPartners described a business intelligence framework that was designed to improve quality outcomes, enhance patient satisfaction, and deliver care more efficiently at a lower cost per encounter. Health-Partners developed an online clinic called "Virtuwell." This 24/7 virtual clinic, which was staffed by nurse practitioners, opened in 2010. It treated 40 different types of routine nonurgent conditions. After treating 40,000 patients via the virtual clinic, they ran the numbers. HealthPartners calculated that they had saved an impressive $88 per episode, the outcomes were determined to be clinically effective, and the satisfaction rates were an enviable 98%!

DISCUSSION QUESTIONS

1. The virtual clinic was created in response to a complex problem of reducing the cost of care per encounter. In this case, HealthPartners saved $88 per encounter by treating common conditions via an online clinic. The savings resulted from more efficient use of resources and enhanced throughput. For the complex problem of reducing the cost of care for each encounter, what other ideas, tactics, or approaches could be used?

2. Imagine that within your organization you and your team came up with the virtual clinic idea. Would you encounter pockets of resistance? How would you work within your own system and use your quality improvement process to move this idea from conception to implementation?

3. The case study of the virtual clinic represents how innovation can foster breakthroughs in cost reduction and quality improvement. Imagine if someone were to create an innovation scale that scored an organization's position from a low of "dull," with little or no innovation," to "sharp," highly innovative. Where would your organization land? Also, do you think nurses should be leaders or followers in fostering a spirit of innovation?

References

Agency for Healthcare Research and Quality. (2012). Enabling patient-centered care through health information. Retrieved from http://www.ahrq.gov/research/findings/evidence-based-reports/er206-abstract.html#Report

Berwick, D. M., Nolan, T. W., & Whittington, J. (2008). The triple aim: Care, health, and cost. *Health Affairs, 27*(3), 759–769.

Boehler, R. (2012, December 4). Translating meaningful use into meaningful outcomes: The key role of clinicians [Webinar]. MedeAnalytics. Retrieved from http://www.medeanalytics.com/cpi

Courneya, P. T., Palattao, K. J., & Gallagher, J. M. (2013). Health-Partners' online clinic for simple conditions delivers savings of $88 per episode and high patient approval. *Health Affairs, 32*(2), 385–392. Retrieved from http://content.healthaffairs.org/content/32/2/385.abstract

Ferguson, J. (2013, January 30). *Achieving the vision of safer and higher quality care.* Retrieved from http://iheusa.org/docs/JamieFerguson.pdf

Institute of Medicine. (2012). Best care at lower cost: The path to continuously learning health care in America. Retrieved from http://www.iom.edu/Reports/2012/Best-Care-at-Lower-Cost-The-Path-to-Continuously-Learning-Health-Care-in-America.aspx

Johnson, L., & Browne, P. (2012, October 18). *Health information technology: IMPACT program overview.* Retrieved from http://www.tenethealth.com/Investors/Documents/Investor%20Presentations/OctoberHealthITInvestorWebinar-October182012.pdf

Organisation for Economic Cooperation and Development. (2009). Health statistics. Retrieved from http://www.oecd.org/health/health-systems/oecdhealthdata2013-frequentlyrequesteddata.htm

World Health Organization. (2014). Health financing. Retrieved from http://gamapserver.who.int/gho/interactive_charts/health_financing/atlas.html

© Leksustuss/Shutterstock, Inc

CHAPTER **11**

Interprofessional Healthcare Teams

Christine Pintz, PhD, RN, FNP-BC, and Jean Johnson, PhD, RN, FAAN

Learning Objectives

At the completion of this chapter, you will be able to:

1. Describe the development and dynamics of interprofessional healthcare teams.
2. Discuss the benefits and challenges of interprofessional healthcare teams.
3. Examine the different types and functions of interprofessional teams.
4. Apply models of interprofessional education to nursing education.

A great deal of attention has been given to the importance of teamwork in health care. Teams are used by many disciplines and can be described as people working together toward a specific goal. Increased emphasis on teamwork in health care has been proposed to create greater efficiency and improve quality. Teams bring together members with diverse talents to manage specific tasks, and effective team dynamics must develop or the team may not be successful. Teams can increase productivity and employee satisfaction, but their success depends on the design and function of the team. Through research and practice, elements that make teams successful have been identified. This text assists the reader in understanding the benefits and challenges of working in teams through case studies focusing on aspects of teamwork in health care.

Interprofessional Teams in Health Care

The idea of interprofessional teams in health care has existed for several decades (Baldwin, 2007; Baldwin & Baldwin, 2007; Grant & Finocchio, 1995). The Institute of Medicine (IOM) released three publications on healthcare quality and patient safety that promoted the importance of highly effective teams in healthcare delivery (Institute of Medicine [IOM], 2000, 2001, 2003). The Institute for Health Care Improvement interprofessional professional education collaborative focused on restructuring health professional education across professions to improve education related to quality and safety (Headrick et al., 1996). Building off the IOM report on competencies for health professions, the Quality and Safety Education for Nurses (QSEN) project incorporated interprofessional education as one of six areas to improve patient care quality (Cronenwett et al., 2007).

WHAT IS AN INTERPROFESSIONAL HEALTHCARE TEAM?

According to Katzenbach and Smith (1993), a team is a set of individuals who exist within a larger group, who come together to work for a particular goal, and who are mutually accountable to each other. To be successful, teams must become interdependent and develop a collective identity that is shared by team members. Interprofessional teams gather together individuals from different professions and disciplines to bring multiple perspectives about solving problems or taking on specific tasks. An interprofessional healthcare team (IHCT) is a group of healthcare professionals who come from different fields within health care. IHCT members must combine their expertise to work in coordinated ways to benefit patients. Teams in health care serve an important role when problems or issues are complex and the solution must come from the perspectives of a diverse set of individuals.

IHCTs experience unique challenges. As members of interprofessional teams, healthcare professionals must go beyond the coordination of healthcare activities. Members of ICHTs also must move past their alignment with their own profession to becoming part of a group that has shared goals and vision. Decisions need be made by the team and not by individual members who share the decisions with the team (Cooper, Dewe, & O'Driscoll, 2001).

LEADERSHIP IN INTERPROFESSIONAL TEAMS

To determine who the leader of the team is, the team must consider a number of points. The team must be clear about what its function is, what the goals and outcomes are, how much support it will receive to accomplish its goals, and who the best person is to facilitate the team's activities. Leaders may be selected or may emerge through the group's work. Leadership can be formal or informal depending on the type of team and the team goal. Some groups have a designated leader at the start, whereas some leaders are selected by the team. Leadership can be shared by group members and be based on the expertise of the team member and the work that needs to be accomplished. The complexity of interprofessional team problems and issues makes it unlikely that a single person can perform all leadership functions. Increasingly, IHCTs are moving toward shared leadership to address the leadership needs of the team. Shared leadership must emerge over time as the team interacts and identifies each team member's expertise.

EFFECT OF INTERPROFESSIONAL TEAMS ON HEALTH PROFESSIONAL SATISFACTION

The team literature suggests that individuals who work in teams have a higher level of work satisfaction (Chuang, Dill, Morgan, & Konrad, 2012; Wamsley et al., 2012). But do interprofessional healthcare teams have increased satisfaction? Flin and Maran

(2004) determined that improved teamwork and communication are described by healthcare workers as among the most important factors in improving clinical effectiveness and job satisfaction. Lemieux-Charles and McGuire (2006) found that collaboration, conflict resolution, and participation predicted satisfaction and perceived team effectiveness.

EFFECT OF INTERPROFESSIONAL TEAMS ON HEALTHCARE OUTCOMES

There has been an increase in research studying the effect of interprofessional teams on the processes and outcomes of health care. Research has been limited by a number of factors. Often the composition of the teams and types of outcomes in studies are operationalized differently, which makes it difficult to synthesize findings across studies. In addition, often the sample sizes are not large, making it difficult to see differences. Moreover, the team rather than the individual is often the unit of analysis, thereby reducing the sample size and leading to underpowered studies.

One aspect that seems to have a large impact on team effectiveness is a diversity of clinical expertise. The multiple perspectives of individuals from a diverse set of disciplines help teams tackle complex problems. This may be based on the team's understanding of the situation and context. In addition, the team is able to draw upon a wide range of expertise (Lemieux-Charles & McGuire, 2006).

Zwarenstein, Goldman, and Reeves (2009) conducted a systematic review to determine how interprofessional collaboration affected the quality of health care. They found, overall, the studies led to an improvement in patient care. However, the review was limited by the small number of studies. They indicated that further studies were needed to determine whether interprofessional collaboration had a significant impact on patient care quality.

Bosch and colleagues (2009) were interested in the role of clinical expertise on the coordination of teamwork and the outcomes of care. They found that clinical expertise was associated with increased team performance but that it had only a mixed effect on team outcomes. Coordinated teams had a better impact on team outcomes but no impact on resource utilization and cost. Clinical expertise and coordination combined had only a small effect on patient outcomes.

The following case studies demonstrate how group processes and dynamics work in IHCTs. **Table 11-1** lists resources that can be used to answer the discussion questions. **Tables 11-2**, **11-3**, and **11-4** provide additional resources.

TABLE 11-1   Resources on Teamwork

Topic	Resource
Competency-based resources for nurses	Quality and Safety Education for Nurses (QSEN). http://www.qsen.org
Continuous quality improvement	Neuhauser, D., Myhre, S., & Alem F. (2004). *Personal continuous quality improvement work book*. Retrieved from http://www.a4hi.org/Education/eduQIWB.cfm
Interprofessional collaborative practice	Interprofessional Education Collaborative. (2011a). *Core competencies for interprofessional collaborative practice: Report of an expert panel*. Washington, DC: Author. Retrieved from http://www.aacn.nche.edu/education-resources/ipecreport.pdf
Interprofessional education	Interprofessional Education Collaborative. (2011b). *Team-based competencies: Building a shared foundation for education and clinical practice* [Conference proceedings]. Retrieved from http://www.aacn.nche.edu/education-resources/IPECProceedings.pdf
Interprofessional education and collaborative practice	World Health Organization. (2010). *Framework for action on interprofessional education and collaborative practice*. Retrieved from http://whqlibdoc.who.int/hq/2010/WHO_HRH_HPN_10.3_eng.pdf?ua=1
Interprofessional team resources	Academy for Healthcare Improvement. (n.d.). Education resources: Working in interdisciplinary teams. Retrieved from http://www.a4hi.org/education/eduWIT.cfm

(Continued)

TABLE 11-1 *(Continued)*

Topic	Resource
Patient-centered care	Stanton, M. W. (2002). Expanding patient-centered care to empower patients and assist providers (AHRQ Publication No. 02-0024). *Research in Action*, 5. Rockville, MD: Agency for Healthcare Research and Quality. Retrieved from http://www.ahrq.gov/research/findings/factsheets/patient-centered/ria-issue5/index.html
Plan-Do-Study-Act (PDSA) cycle	Institute for Health Care Improvement. (2011). Plan-Do-Study-Act (PDSA) worksheet. Retrieved from http://www.ihi.org/knowledge/Pages/Tools/PlanDoStudyActWorksheet.aspx
Professional communication and team collaboration	O'Donnell, M., & Rosenstein, A. H. (2008, April). Professional communication and team collaboration. In *Patient safety and quality: An evidence-based handbook for nurses* (AHRQ Publication No. 08-0043). Rockville, MD: Agency for Healthcare Research and Quality. Retrieved from http://www.ncbi.nlm.nih.gov/books/NBK2637/
Situation-Background-Assessment-Recommendation (SBAR)	Institute for Health Care Improvement. (2011). SBAR technique for communication: A situational briefing model. Retrieved from http://www.ihi.org/resources/Pages/Tools/SBARTechniqueforCommunicationASituationalBriefingModel.aspx
TeamSTEPPS	Agency for Healthcare Research and Quality. (2008). *Pocket guide: TeamSTEPPS. Strategies and tools to enhance performance and patient safety* (AHRQ Publication No. 06-0020-2). Rockville, MD: Author. Retrieved from http://www.ahrq.gov/professionals/education/curriculum-tools/teamstepps/instructor/essentials/pocketguide.pdf

TABLE 11-2 Team Development

Stage of Team Development	Characteristics
Tuckman's Model of Stages of Small-Group Development	
Forming	The team forms and begins the process of setting goals. Team members begin to learn how to work together.
Storming	Team members develop and vie for roles within the group. Conflict develops between individuals and subgroups. Teams must resolve conflict in order to develop shared vision and build trust.

Stage of Team Development	Characteristics
Tuckman's Model of Stages of Small-Group Development	
Norming	The team begins to address the task. Now that conflict is resolved, there is agreement, acceptance, and consensus among team members for team roles and decisions.
Performing	During this stage, the focus is on achieving team goals. The team has developed an identity and has learned how to work together.
Adjourning	This is the process of ending the team after the goal has been achieved.
Drinka's Model of Healthcare Teamwork	
Forming	Team members function according to their profession's perspective. IHCTs often ignore conflict and move to the norming phase before establishing clear goals.
Norming	Conflict is suppressed. Leadership doesn't always coincide with expertise or time limitations. Competition between disciplines may occur. Team members may compete because roles overlap. Conflict may become difficult to manage.
Confronting	Conflict is addressed. Teams can manage conflict by engaging in problem solving and constructive confrontation. Informal leaders may emerge. Groups that cannot manage conflict may return to the norming phase. Well-functioning teams move to the next phase through effective collaboration.
Performing	Team is performing well when focus is on team development and performance and not on individual members. In addition, the individual characteristics of the team members become an asset rather than a liability.
Leaving	Interdisciplinary teams generally have turnover. Leaving may be temporary or permanent, and it may involve one or more members of the team. The team may move through previous phases as members come and go.

Sources: Data from Tuckman, B. W., & Jensen, M. A. (1977). Stages of small-group development revisited. *Group and Organization Studies, 2,* 419–427; and Drinka, T. J. K., & Clark, P. G. (2000). *Healthcare teamwork: Interdisciplinary practice and teaching.* Westport, CT: Auburn House.

TABLE 11-3 Team Types

Team Type	Characteristics
Crews	Crews are highly structured and well defined. Team roles are prescribed and short-term goals are shared. Examples of this type of team are surgical teams, cockpit crews, and sports teams.
Task forces	Task forces' tasks are unstructured and roles of the team members are loosely defined. The goal is clear at the outset, but how to accomplish the goal is not. Task forces form with the task defined and work to develop a plan to achieve the goal.
Standing or functional teams	Standing or functional teams have many tasks to complete and no clear way to accomplish them. Standing teams need to work together for the long term, so being able to work together is essential. Examples of this type of team are curriculum committees and quality improvement committees.

Source: Data from Kline, T. (1999). *Remaking teams: The revolutionary research-based guide that puts theory into practice.* San Francisco, CA: Jossey-Bass.

TABLE 11-4 Characteristics of Effective Teams

Clear goals and objectives
Results-driven structure
Competent team members
Unified commitment
Collaborative climate
High standards
External support and encouragement
Principled leadership

Source: Data from Larson, C. E., & LaFasto, F. M. J. (1989). *Teamwork: What must go right, what can go wrong.* Newbury Park, CA: Sage.

CASE STUDY: *Valley View Health Care*

Dr. Bill Smith recently sold his private solo family practice to a hospital corporation. The medical corporation is planning to develop the practice into a medical home, and the practice will be called Valley View Health Care. A patient-centered medical home (PCMH) is a type of healthcare practice that is composed of several elements. Health care should be patient-centered and culturally competent. PCMHs develop a partnership between healthcare providers and patients and their families. The health care provided is more efficient and effective by incorporating information technology, quality improvement, and evidence-based practice.

Dr. Smith has been in practice for 25 years, and he employs a family nurse practitioner, Gretchen Wilson, who has worked for the practice for 12 years. Ms. Wilson's practice has mainly focused on elderly patients, and she follows all the practice's nursing home patients. The practice will merge with a surgical practice that consists of a general surgeon, Dr. Ellen Davis, and a physician assistant, Steve Elliott. The hospital corporation will add an endocrinologist, a certified diabetic nurse educator, and a nurse manager who will manage the day-to-day clinical activities and will develop and implement the quality improvement program. They are thinking of adding another provider but are unsure whether it should be a physician, physician assistant, or nurse practitioner. The hospital corporation has added an electronic health record (EHR) and all the providers are required to use it. The office will have two locations about 10 miles apart. The city office is close to the hospital, and the other office is located in an outlying suburb. As these two practices merge and as new employees are added, this healthcare team will face some challenges.

DISCUSSION QUESTIONS

1. Describe the characteristics of an interprofessional healthcare team. How does the World Health Organization define interprofessional collaborative practice?

2. What are some attributes of successful healthcare teams?

3. According to Tuckman (1965; Tuckman & Jensen, 1977), teams go through stages as they develop. (See Table 11-2.) What are those stages and what are the characteristics of each stage?

4. What stage of development is this team in? Why do you think so?

5. What are some of the challenges this team will encounter in the formation process?

As these two practices consolidate, several issues have emerged. The hospital corporation has asked Dr. Smith to serve as the medical director for the new practice. As he assumes his leadership role, he begins to assess how the practice is currently functioning. In addition, he begins to develop new policies for the practice. He has determined that all of the providers will work at both offices. He has also determined that Mr. Elliott, who has primarily worked in surgical settings, will also see primary care patients. Dr. Smith feels this is necessary, at this time, in order to provide care to all of the primary care patients and to help the practice grow. In time, he plans to add another primary care provider, though he has not discussed this with Mr. Elliott.

Dr. Smith's new policies are affecting Ms. Wilson. She has been working at the office in the suburban location. Most of her nursing home clients are located near that office. In addition, she has been able to schedule patients around the times that she has to pick up and drop off her children at school. She is not sure how she will manage working in both offices. Dr. Davis also has some concerns about the changes occurring in the practice. Her old practice did not have an EHR, and she is uncomfortable with the new technology. She has been having her assistant input information into the EHR for her. This has led to a reduction in income because the assistant is not coding visits correctly.

DISCUSSION QUESTIONS

1. What stage is this team entering? Why?
2. How can this team manage its progress through the stages? What are some strategies that the team can use to minimize or resolve conflict?
3. Dr. Smith has been selected as the leader of this team. What role will the leader play with this team? What are the challenges he will experience as this team begins to work together? How should he deal with these challenges?

The Valley View Health team has been working together for about 6 months. They seem to get along pretty well and have resolved the issues previously described. Dr. Smith decided that he needed input from the team on how the new policies should be implemented. They meet monthly to discuss the practice and how problems should be solved. Mr. Elliott has agreed to see primary care patients once a week to help with the patient load. The team reviewed the revenue and expenses and decided to employ a new primary care provider in the next year. The new provider will work at the city office, leaving Ms. Wilson to work primarily at the suburban office. She has been able to juggle her children's transportation needs with her husband and her mother. Dr. Davis went to a training course on the electronic medical record system and has had no further problems using the system.

The members of the team have been happy with Dr. Smith's leadership. He has been open to input from the team and has worked with team members to solve problems associated with the new practice. He has had several of the members lead initiatives based on their interest and expertise. Dr. Smith has been enjoying his new role as administrator and has decided to pursue a master's in health administration. He is currently taking an organizational development course and is learning about team development and process. He thinks that the team is starting to work well together but believes that they have not developed a team identity.

DISCUSSION QUESTIONS

1. What stage of team development is the Valley View Health group in? What are the specific characteristics that point to the stage?

2. What are some strategies that will enable Dr. Smith to promote team identity and cohesiveness? How will the group develop shared vision and goals?

The team at Valley View Health Care has begun reviewing how they perform. Although the practice has been successful, they are interested in identifying some ways that the practice can earn additional revenue. At their monthly team meeting, they began to brainstorm about ideas. Mr. Elliott suggests that they start offering cosmetic procedures. A new member of the team, Dr. Mark Phillips, a family practice physician, suggests they add some complementary medicine practitioners to the practice. Dr. Smith is interested in seeing whether expanding the practice to add another office would increase revenue. They decide to form a subcommittee of the group to look into these ideas.

In addition, the practice has hired Martha Hilliard as the new nurse manager. She has a background in hospital quality improvement and oversees the practice's quality improvement program. She has begun looking at the practice's data and its adherence to the Healthcare Effectiveness Data and Information Set (HEDIS) measures. She plans to review the practice's adherence to the Comprehensive Diabetic Performance Measures. Her preliminary analysis has found the practice's rate is 70%. She knows that this is below the national average. She plans to work with the members of the management team to identify ways to improve the practice's performance.

DISCUSSION QUESTIONS

1. There are typically three types of teams. What are the different types of teams and what are the unique characteristics of each? What type of team will the Valley View Health team form? What makes you think so?

2. What are some important characteristics of a team in the performing stage?

3. How will the group determine which revenue-producing strategies should be implemented? Should a new team be formed? What type of team should be formed?

4. There are a number of models of quality improvement. Describe the Plan-Do-Study-Act (PDSA) method. How might Valley View Health implement a continuous quality improvement (CQI) program? How should Ms. Hilliard lead the team in this effort?

A year has passed and the team is conducting their first leadership retreat. There have been some changes to the team. Ms. Wilson's husband has been transferred, and so she will be leaving the practice in a month. Dr. Davis will be transitioning off the team because her surgical practice is very busy and she doesn't have time. A new nurse practitioner has been with the practice for 6 months. There is a plan to add another primary care physician to the practice in the next year.

The team decides to focus on improving its adherence to performance measures. It decides to target measures where adherence is less than 75%. The practice has improved its performance on the diabetes measures. It will use the retreat to discuss which measures to target next year. It will also discuss the three revenue-producing ideas and select one to develop. A subcommittee was formed to review the ideas, and they will present their findings. The team will also discuss who to add to the team to replace the members who have left. At this point, the team reflects on the successes and challenges they have experienced in the last year. All of the team members feel ready to develop goals for the next year.

DISCUSSION QUESTIONS

1. What stage of team development is the Valley View Health team in at this point? What is your rationale for your selection?

2. Is the Valley View Health team effective? What makes you think so?

3. What are some challenges that this team may experience in the future? How can the team address these challenges?

Team Communication

Team communication is an essential component for effective teamwork. Moreover, effective communication leads to higher quality health care and better patient safety. But professionals who come from different healthcare disciplines may not always communicate in an effective manner.

CASE STUDY: *Pinehurst Hospital Operating Room*

Dr. Adam Heller is the chief anesthesiologist at a university-affiliated hospital. Lately, he has been noticing that things have not been running smoothly in the operating room (OR). He has noticed that cases are not starting on time and the operating rooms are not turning over as efficiently as they have in the past. The OR nurse manager, Ann Hayes, has told him that she is concerned about excess staffing costs because of the delayed throughput. They wonder if there is a solution to the problem.

The nurse manager is in a master's program and is learning about different models of team communication. She shares some articles with Dr. Heller so that they can discuss the models and select an appropriate approach to improving the OR team's performance. They identify two models: the TeamSTEPPS program and the Situation-Background-Assessment-Recommendation (SBAR) technique.

DISCUSSION QUESTIONS

1. Why might TeamSTEPPS be a good approach for dealing with the OR issues? How does it contrast with the SBAR approach? Why might SBAR be a better approach?

2. What challenges would they encounter if they implemented TeamSTEPPS? What challenges would they encounter implementing SBAR?

3. How should Dr. Heller and Ms. Hayes gain organizational support for TeamSTEPPS or SBAR? How should they gain support from the members of the OR team?

4. Based on your responses to the previous questions, what method should be selected? Explain your rationale.

The OR team have begun to implement their new program. They have been able to improve communication between OR staff and the anesthesiology group but have had difficulty getting the surgeons involved with the program. The OR staff and physicians feel that the OR is running more smoothly. However, when examining the data, Ms. Hayes finds that there has been only a slight improvement in OR turnover time and throughput. Two factors seem to be responsible for the lack of improvement: Surgeons are late, which delays start time, and patients do not arrive to the OR on time.

DISCUSSION QUESTIONS

1. How does this new team provide situation monitoring?
2. Give some examples of how this team provides mutual support.
3. Are there examples of clear and accurate communication? If so, what are they?
4. How will this group involve all the stakeholders in the change process. What are some strategies that could be used to get the surgeons and other hospital departments involved in improving turnover time and throughput?

Interprofessional Education

Health professional collaboration has become a focus for policymakers because of the potential for reduction of error, better care coordination, and improved patient safety. The increasing complexity of health care makes it difficult for a single healthcare professional to be responsible for all aspects of care. However, healthcare professionals are often not prepared to work in teams when caring for patients. Institutions that educate health professional students must begin to develop programs that prepare their graduates for teamwork in the healthcare environment.

CASE STUDY: *Lakeside College*

Faculty representing several health professional education programs have formed a committee whose purpose is to increase interprofessional education experiences. The committee was formed because the new university provost wants the school to promote interprofessional collaboration.

There had been several programs at his previous university. Members of the committee are two nursing faculty, three medical school faculty, one social work faculty, one physician assistant program faculty, and two healthcare management faculty. Several of the faculty are veterans of other committees created to promote interprofessional education in the past. These initiatives have not been successful. They plan to develop a class on patient-centered care. They have had several meetings but are no closer to developing the course. The major challenge is finding a time in the schedules of the different educational programs for the students to meet. In addition, there is disagreement about what should be taught in the class and what type of interprofessional team skills the course should promote.

DISCUSSION QUESTIONS

1. How should the committee begin the planning process?
2. What resources should they identify when developing this program?
3. What challenges might they experience in developing this program?
4. Identify the core competencies developed by the Interprofessional Education Collaborative (IEC) and discuss how they could be integrated into the proposed course.
5. The report *Team-Based Competencies: Building a Shared Foundation for Education and Clinical Practice* (Interprofessional Education Collaborative, 2011b) identified restraining factors that prevent interprofessional activities in education. What restraining factors are present in this case? How can these restraining factors be overcome?
6. What educational approaches could be developed in your own educational program that would support interprofessional education? Discuss how you would benefit from having an interprofessional education experience.

Conclusion

Health care is increasingly moving toward focusing healthcare delivery on IHCTs. Although the development of IHCTs can be challenging, bringing together individuals with diverse talents, developing the team to incorporate proper team dynamics, and providing the appropriate resources can help to make the team successful. Teams can increase productivity and employee satisfaction. Research to identify aspects of teamwork that lead to better patient outcomes still needs to be done. Current studies do show that there are benefits to IHCTs.

References

Agency for Healthcare Research and Quality. (2008). *Pocket guide: TeamSTEPPS. strategies and tools to enhance performance and patient safety* (AHRQ Publication No. 06-0020-2). Rockville, MD: Author.

Baldwin, D. C., Jr. (2007). Some historical notes on interdisciplinary and interprofessional education and practice in health care in the USA. 1996. *Journal of Interprofessional Care, 21*(Suppl. 1), 23–37.

Baldwin, D. C., Jr., & Baldwin, M. A. (2007). Interdisciplinary education and health team training: A model for learning and service. 1979. *Journal of Interprofessional Care, 21*(Suppl. 1), 52–69.

Bosch, M., Faber, M. J., Cruijsberg, J., Voerman, G., Letherman,, S., Grol, P. T. M., ... Wensing, M. (2009). Effectiveness of patient care teams and the role of clinical expertise and coordination: A literature review. *Medical Care Research and Review, 66,* 5S–35S. doi:10.1177/1077558709343295

Chuang, E., Dill, J., Morgan, J. C., & Konrad, T. R. (2012). A configurational approach to the relationship between high-performance work practices and frontline health care worker outcomes. *Health Services Research, 47*(4), 1460–1481.

Cooper, C. L., Dewe, P. J., & O'Driscoll, M. P. (2001). *Organizational stress: A review and critique of theory, research and applications.* Thousand Oaks, CA: Sage.

Cronenwett, L., Sherwood, G., Barnsteiner, J., Disch, J., Johnson, J., Mitchell, P., ... Warren, J. (2007). Quality and safety education for nurses. *Nursing Outlook, 55*(3), 122–131.

Flin, R., & Maran, N. (2004). Identifying and training non-technical skills in acute medicine. *Quality and Safety in Health Care, 13*(Suppl. I), 180–184.

Grant, R. W., & Finocchio, L. J. (1995). *Interdisciplinary collaborative teams in primary care: A model curriculum and resource guide*. San Francisco, CA: Pew Health Profession Commission.

Headrick, L. A., Knapp, M., Neuhauser, D., Gelmon, S., Norman, L., Quinn, D., & Baker, R. (1996). Working from upstream to improve health care: The IHI interdisciplinary professional education collaborative. *Joint Commission Journal on Quality Improvement, 22*, 149–164.

Institute of Medicine. (2000). *To err is human: Building a safer health system*. Washington, DC: National Academy Press.

Institute of Medicine. (2001). *Crossing the quality chasm: A new health system for the 21st century*. Washington, DC: National Academy Press.

Institute of Medicine. (2003). *Keeping patients safe: Transforming the work environment for nurses*. Washington, DC: National Academy Press.

Interprofessional Education Collaborative. (2011a). *Core competencies for interprofessional collaborative practice: Report of an expert panel*. Washington, DC: Author.

Interprofessional Education Collaborative. (2011b, February 16–17). *Team-based competencies: Building a shared foundation for education and clinical practice* [Conference Proceedings]. Retrieved from http://www.aacn.nche.edu/leading-initiatives/IPECProceedings.pdf

Katzenbach, J. R., & Smith, D. K. (1993). *The wisdom of teams: Creating the high-performance organization*. Boston, MA: Harvard Business School.

Kline, T. (1999). *Remaking teams: The revolutionary research-based guide that puts theory into practice*. San Francisco, CA: Jossey-Bass.

Larson, C. E., & LaFasto, F. M. J. (1989). *Teamwork: What must go right, what can go wrong*. Newberry Park, CA: Sage.

Lemieux-Charles, L., & McGuire, W. L. (2006). What do we know about health care team effectiveness? A review of the literature. *Medical Care Research and Review, 63*, 263–300. doi:10.1177/1077558706287003

O'Donnell, M., & Rosenstein, A. H. (2008, April). Professional communication and team collaboration. In *Patient safety and quality: An evidence-based handbook for nurses* (AHRQ Publication No. 08-0043). Rockville, MD: Agency for Healthcare Research and Quality.

Tuckman, B. W. (1965). Developmental sequence in small groups. *Psychology Bulletin, 63*, 384–399.

Tuckman, B. W., & Jensen, M. A. (1977). Stages of small-group development revisited. *Group and Organization Studies, 2*, 419–427.

Wamsley, M., Staves, J., Kroon, L., Topp, K., Hossaini, M., Newlin, B., … O'Brien, B. (2012). The impact of an interprofessional standardized patient exercise on attitudes toward working in interprofessional teams. *Journal of Interprofessional Care, 26*(1), 28–35.

Zwarenstein, M., Goldman, J., & Reeves, S. (2009). Interprofessional collaboration: Effects of practice-based interventions on professional practice and healthcare outcomes. *Cochrane Database of Systematic Reviews*, (3), CD000072. doi:10.1002/14651858.CD000072.pub2

CHAPTER 12

The Clinical Nurse Leader

Pamela Abraham, MSN, RN, CNL, Catherine Edmonds, MSN, RN, CNL, Jennifer Kareivis, MSN, RN, CNL, and Marianne Sweeney, MSN, RN, CNL

Do not go where the path may lead, go instead where there is no path and leave a trail.

—Ralph Waldo Emerson

Learning Objectives

At the completion of this chapter, you will be able to:

1. Identify how Clinical Nurse Leaders (CNLs) influence practice at the microsystem level.
2. Apply evidence-based practice guidelines to improve care outcomes.
3. Demonstrate how CNLs affect quality of practice and cost outcomes.
4. Illustrate the leadership role of the CNL in clinical decision making.

---

*Unless a citation is provided, examples in this chapter are drawn from real situations experienced by or known to the authors.

5. Respect the attributes that members of intra- and interdisciplinary teams bring to patient care.

6. Discuss the role of the CNL in care accountability.

"Nursing, as the most trusted profession, is in a central and unique position to redesign the complex and fragmented patient care delivery system that currently exists" (Tornabeni, 2006, p. 4). Healthcare challenges in the twenty-first century include patients with multiple chronic conditions, an aging and diverse population, health disparities, and limited English proficiency. Reports released by the Institute of Medicine, Robert Wood Johnson Foundation, and American Hospital Association all cite the need to make changes in healthcare delivery and the education of health professionals to improve patient outcomes.

The nursing profession is versatile and well respected, and it has the opportunity to educate innovators to address these challenges. One new role for nurses that highlights their potential as innovators is the Clinical Nurse Leader (CNL), an advanced generalist clinician role designed to improve clinical and cost outcomes for specific groups of patients at the microsystem level. Charged with coordinating care and in some cases actively providing direct care in complex situations, the CNL has the responsibility for translating and applying research findings to design, implement, and evaluate plans of care for patients (Institute of Medicine [IOM], 2011). This new transformational nursing role, the first in 40 years, has been adopted by the Veterans Affairs (VA) system, among others. According to Cathy Rick, chief nursing officer of the Department of Veteran Affairs, the VA intends to employ CNLs in all of its medical centers by 2016 (Office of Nursing Services, 2009).

The CNL role was developed by the American Association of Colleges of Nursing (AACN) in collaboration with leaders from the education and practice arenas. Two AACN task forces were convened to identify (1) how to improve the quality of patient care and (2) how to best prepare nurses with the competencies needed to thrive in the current and future healthcare system (Tornabeni, 2006). AACN (2007) developed a white paper that serves as a resource to guide the multifaceted role of the CNL.

Various roles of the CNL include lateral integrator, clinician, outcomes manager, information/data manager, educator, patient/family advocate, team manager, systems/risk analyst, member of a profession, and lifelong learner. Additionally, the CNL is a reflective practitioner, noticing patterns from within a systems perspective. This chapter will explore the ways in which these roles combine to make significant changes in a complex environment at the microsystem level. Examples of situations in which CNL initiatives could result in an improved outcome for patients and families, as well as real-world examples of such initiatives, are interwoven throughout the chapter.

A Day in the Life

Daily activities of the CNL include an initial unit environmental screen, which includes activities such as checking the hallway for accurate signage and clutter reduction to foster ease of passage for transport of patients. Defective equipment is sent to the Biomedical department for repair. A daily census is obtained and reviewed for new admissions and transfers. Reports on the condition of each patient on the unit from each staff nurse identify potential issues and safety concerns. Indwelling devices are reviewed for medical necessity, or their discontinuation is discussed. Attention is given to asking about each patient's skin condition to assess for risk for developing hospital-acquired pressure ulcers. Every patient's chart is reviewed for history and physical information, testing related to diagnosis, core measure review, and additional consultations that may benefit the patient's outcomes, such as physical therapy, palliative care, or a visit from the chaplain.

CNL Framework

COMMUNICATION

The CNL integrates care by facilitating communication between disciplines while addressing frontline issues in real time. For instance, a CNL may call the Information Systems department to resolve computer hardware and documentation issues. Perhaps prescribers had trouble finding orthostatic vital signs in the computer. The CNL would then call Information Systems, and as a result, a separate tab in the computer would be created for "orthostatic blood pressures," which is a huge prescriber satisfier. The separate tab also would be safer for patients because the doctors and physician assistants are then readily able to identify the orthostatic blood pressures.

A CNL also calls prescribers to speak with families or patients who have questions. Safe discharge transitions are fostered by a discussion of postdischarge arrangements with the patient care manager, social worker, or home care coordinator. For example, a CNL may learn that a patient lives alone, has no family nearby, and uses a walker. In addition, physical therapy staff may have identified that this patient is deconditioned and would benefit by a short stay in a subacute rehabilitation facility. Aware of these issues, the CNL can alert the patient care manager and social worker about a possible patient discharge to a local rehabilitation facility so that they can look into availability.

A CNL's daily rounds on each patient are an opportunity for interactive communication with patients and families regarding the patient's condition. During rounds, education and safety information, infection prevention, and plan of care are reviewed so all stakeholders can be engaged. A CNL will have a conversation with each patient daily about his or her diagnosis, new medications, new procedures, and measures to prevent infection to make sure patients and family members are aware of what the plan of care entails.

Communicating with the various disciplines and the patient is a big part of the CNL role. For example, patients have mentioned to CNLs that they may not want certain treatments, or they are "tired of being in the hospital." Sometimes patients do not feel comfortable confiding in their families their true wishes for the plan of care. A CNL can step in, speak with a doctor about a patient's wishes, and arrange meetings with the families so that the patient's wishes for care can be voiced and honored.

DISCUSSION QUESTIONS

1. Describe how the CNL demonstrates patient and community advocacy.
2. How does the CNL facilitate lateral integration between the various disciplines?
3. Describe how CNLs have the opportunity to foster communication with each patient.
4. Describe the value of the CNL's continuity of care in the acute care setting.
5. Identify how rounding fosters communication and patient engagement.

INTERDISCIPLINARY CARE

Interdisciplinary discharge planning rounds occur biweekly to review patients' prognoses and their courses of stay, and also to plan for a safe transition upon release from the acute care environment. These rounds help the team identify the plan of care and, if indicated, allocate resources, such as physical therapy or occupational therapy.

During CNL role immersion, CNLs meet with various departments within the hospital, including finance, quality, risk management, social work, patient safety, palliative care, infection preventionists, and wound care. These meetings provide the basis for creation of vital relationships between CNLs and diverse disciplines. For example, during an initial meeting with the Finance department, a CNL can be educated about reimbursement and other financial aspects of their organization. Understanding care from this perspective enables a CNL to recognize possible cost-saving initiatives. Connecting a person with the Finance department fosters the reciprocal relationship.

The patient-centered interdisciplinary team is available for consultation during the hospital stay as the need arises. For example, in one such meeting, a CNL spent some time in the Senior Services department observing an outpatient geriatric assessment given by the Senior Services social worker and the geriatrician. An in-depth assessment was completed for the patient and the patient's family situation. The purpose of the assessment was to assist the patient and family with community resources and needs in the home. Observing this assessment process was an opportunity for the CNL to see what the geriatrician assessed in the consultation and to help facilitate the geriatric services involvement with appropriate patients on the units. In this case meeting with the palliative care practitioners also allowed for a better understanding of their contribution to the interdisciplinary team, including development of goals of overall care and not just hospice care.

Another example might be a CNL visiting neighboring subacute rehabilitation facilities. Making such visits during the immersion period adds a contextual connection with those locations. Understanding the environment, the staff, and the functionality helps the CNL prepare patients and families for the transitional phase before they actually go home. By seeing the facilities in the area, the CNL gains a better understanding of the settings for subacute rehabilitation and nursing home placement. With this knowledge, the CNL can then assist patients and families in making choices and navigating the process of transition to a facility. The CNL, along with the social worker, can encourage all families to visit each subacute facility to see where their loved ones may be spending some recuperation time.

In a multifaceted approach to solutions, regular discussion by an interdisciplinary team identifies pertinent issues. On each unit, biweekly discharge rounds and monthly geriatric rounds help resolve issues that may arise during the hospital stay. Patient case studies are presented to the team by staff nurses who have identified issues that need addressing. CNL rounds facilitate communication among all disciplines, which improves patient safety and ensures accurate transfer of information. It is an efficient use of time and resources. CNL rounds promote mutual respect through group problem solving, cohesiveness, and creativity, which are characteristics of a synergistic healthcare team. Nurse satisfaction and autonomy increase because patient concerns can be addressed in real time. An issue identified during geriatric rounds may be as simple as addressing a patient's need to begin a bowel regimen as a result of using narcotic pain relief after a repaired hip fracture. Discussions may also include addressing the level of care of an 85-year-old patient who has undergone emergency surgery for a subdural hematoma and who has not recuperated from surgery as expected.

DISCUSSION QUESTIONS

1. What is the value of meeting with the interdisciplinary team when first beginning your role as a CNL in your organization? Which individuals would be essential to meet and establish relationships with?

2. Give examples of how the interdisciplinary team can improve the patient's hospital experience.

3. Describe how the interdisciplinary team reduces the patient's length of stay.

4. Identify how the interdisciplinary team promotes nurse satisfaction.

MICROSYSTEMS

Healthcare delivery is complex within, between, and across clinical microsystems. Each clinical microsystem must do the work, meet staff needs, and maintain itself as a clinical unit to contribute to the larger organization. Viewing organizations as complex adaptive systems encourages leaders to be flexible and aware of the unpredictability of patients' holistic needs. CNLs dress in business casual and wear a white lab coat. They are visual reminders of safety and they are the "resource" that every discipline in the microsystem seeks for problem-solving techniques and answers.

Working consistent 8-hour shifts, CNLs are a constant presence for the healthcare team, patients, and families. Their steady presence is essential in the care of patients and families. They are Clinical Scene Investigators (CSIs), assessing the environment and identifying and addressing system issues, all while advocating for patients and staff on a daily basis. Continuity by the CNL promotes positive interactive relationships. CNLs promote patient, family, and staff autonomy. CNLs "connect the docs" to link healthcare providers with each other to facilitate communication. The lateral integration is most evident in this role.

Take, for example, a situation in which a diabetic patient is admitted with a wound to his foot caused by a blister from his shoe. After debridement of the wound, the patient needs to have negative pressure wound therapy (NPWT) applied to the site. During the absence of the wound nurse, a CNL can assist in monitoring the wound and NPWT and in changing the dressing to the site. In addition, the patient and his fiancée need to be taught how to change the dressing so that they will be able to do so at home. The CNL will spend time demonstrating to the patient and his fiancée how to change the dressing and care for the wound, and review signs and symptoms of non-healing that need to be reported to the physician. On the day of discharge, the CNL can again review the steps for dressing change and answer any questions the patient and family have. In following up with the physician about the patient's progress, the CNL would like be able to report that the wound showed great improvement and the NPWT would be discontinued.

An important contribution at the microsystem level is that issues pertaining to patients, families, safety, or infection prevention are addressed immediately. This unique role enables CNLs to work alongside the frontline team, identify issues, and resolve them. Lateral integration enables CNLs to assess and determine the best plan of care for the patient and which consultations may be of benefit. No other role is patient- and family-centered in such a comprehensive, holistic way.

CNLs' impact on patient care is becoming more apparent within units and organizations. Accountability for positive patient outcomes is what motivates the CNL to develop initiatives when an issue has been identified, such as an increase in pressure ulcers. These initiatives may include development and implementation of education programs for the nurses and ancillary staff or development of a checklist to ensure certain criteria are met. CNLs within the organization meet monthly to share and celebrate their innovations and positive outcomes. The outcomes are presented in professional publications and at national conferences.

DISCUSSION QUESTIONS

1. What impact or effect does the CNL have in each microsystem?
2. How do the staff nurse and CNL collaborate to improve patient outcomes?
3. How can microsystem changes ultimately affect the macrosystem?
4. What effect does early identification of issues have on patient outcomes?

EVIDENCE-BASED PRACTICE

The CNL has the ability and resources to develop initiatives to prevent errors and improve patient outcomes. CNLs participate in quality improvement strategies, examining resource utilization, mapping current processes, and conducting root cause analyses of adverse events.

Hospital-acquired urinary tract infections can increase the patient's length of stay or require a readmission. A CNL could, for example, collaborate with infection preventionists to develop a device day list that tracks the number of indwelling catheters. The CNL could review the numbers daily for medical indication. In order to prevent contamination, the CNL could also conduct a recent in-service to refresh nursing staff on proper techniques for acquiring specimens. Finally, the CNL could discuss patients with indwelling catheter during the unit's twice-daily briefings when all staff are present.

Prevention of hospital-acquired infections, which also consists of staff hand washing, are paramount foci for the CNLs. To meet this goal, the infection preventionists have an ongoing collaboration with the CNLs. One intervention that was implemented includes visual reminders such a "Wash In Wash Out" signs, which are located on all the automatic soap dispensers.

DISCUSSION QUESTIONS

1. How does the CNL use technology and information to improve patient outcomes?
2. Describe how the CNL can prevent hospital-acquired infections.
3. Identify ways the CNL uses evidence-based practice to reduce hospital-acquired infections.

QUALITY MANAGEMENT

Falls, pressure ulcers, and infection prevention results are reported by individual hospitals and in the National Database of Nursing Quality Indicators (NDNQI). Hospital Consumer Assessment of Healthcare Providers and Systems (HCAHP) produces comparable data of the patient's perspective on care, allowing objective and meaningful comparisons between hospital domains that are important to consumers. Results can create an incentive for hospitals to improve care. Initiatives, such as noise reduction, call backs, and patient education, are then developed based on these results. Important statistics related to Nursing Quality Indicators (NDNQI), for example, falls, pressure ulcers, infection control, are distributed to staff each month in a CNL update. The update highlights the "need to know" topics for RNs on the front lines of patient care. This is another example of a CNL initiative to improve communication among the staff.

The Centers for Medicare and Medicaid Services (CMS) requires core measures in areas such as pneumonia, pain management, congestive heart failure (CHF), acute myocardial infarction (AMI), physician–nurse collaboration, patient satisfaction, and surgical care (Surgical Care Improvement Project, or SCIP). These measures also drive CNL initiatives. For example, in one hospital a CHF education packet was recently developed to enhance patient and family knowledge of this chronic illness. The ultimate goal was to have an educated consumer who follows a safe regimen at home and follows up with a healthcare provider, thus preventing readmission to the hospital. Another example of the CNL's role in promoting compliance with the core measures is antibiotic use within 24 hours of surgical end time. One facility identified multiple cases of postoperative antibiotic administration falling out of the 24-hour window after the surgical end time. In response, CNLs conducted staff education so the staff could recognize the importance of core measures, proper timing of antibiotics, and identification of improper profiling in the Medication Administration Record (MAR). The CNLs review postoperative charts daily to verify appropriate doses were profiled in the MAR and appropriate administration times are listed.

CNLs also conduct and monitor National Patient Safety Goals (NPSG) audits and communicate the results to staff. CNLs develop initiatives if there is a deficiency below 85%. For example, a hand hygiene audit in one hospital revealed a 65% deficiency in hand washing by RNs when entering the patient room. Initiatives taken by the CNLs included discussing the topic at monthly staff meetings and adding more hand-washing dispensers mounted accessibly on the walls of the unit.

In addition to quantitative outcomes, quality of the patient's experience during the hospitalization is equally as important. As a CNL rounds daily on their patients and families, he or she begins to develop a connection through the entire course of a patient's stay. In a complex environment, the pace can be fast and impersonal. A CNL's connection with a patient and his or her family fosters a relationship of active listening, educating, and caring. Recognizing what is important to the patient and family is vital to engage the team in a shared responsibility toward the recovery process. The CNL assists the patient to move more efficiently through the healthcare system, addressing fragmentation of care and gaps in communication and minimizing unnecessary disruptions, delays, and adverse effects.

One CNL led a quality improvement initiative in an acute care setting. Because there were 28 falls in 2009 and 23 in 2010, falls reduction was identified to be a unit priority. Staff in-services were conducted to educate and foster awareness and accountability for each fall.

In 2010, after completing a literature search, a Falls Team was developed as an opportunity to reduce falls. The team, including RNs and patient care assistants, meets monthly to discuss new strategies on fall prevention. Some of the outcomes identified in these meetings were the need for new chair alarms and for patients identified as at risk not to be left alone in the rest room or on a commode at any time.

A team member developed a *Falls Bulletin* that provides staff with a unique account of each fall, circumstances leading up to the fall, cause of the fall, patient outcomes, and prevention strategies. The bulletin is distributed to every staff member to raise awareness about being more vigilant and to remind staff that it is the entire team's responsibility to ensure patient safety.

Because of increased staff awareness and accountability, falls reduction from 23 to 10 in 2011 was a cost savings of approximately $52,000 ($4,000 per fall) (Inouye, Brown, & Tinetti, 2009).

Success at decreasing the falls rate on one unit has led to the other unit's adapting some of the practices developed by the Falls Team, including the *Falls Bulletin*, for its own use. Sustainability of these initiatives is the ongoing challenge.

In another situation, a CNL identified an increase in hospital-acquired pressure ulcers on patients' heels and ulcers due to mechanical devices. In collaboration with the wound care nurse, the CNL presented independent study packets and in-services to the staff throughout the hospital. New heel protectors and soft silicone oxygen tubing were added to the pressure ulcer prevention regimen.

Staff awareness, education, and staff feedback foster high-quality patient care. In this situation, there was a 90% reduction in heel and device-related ulcers as a result of this intervention of staff education and engagement.

In yet another example of a CNL initiative, on a medical floor, an increase in stage 2 ear pressure ulcers was identified in several patients who received oxygen via nasal cannula. When a root cause analysis was done, it was noted that the incidence occurred in a population with sensory perception impairment. The CNL's mission was to find a protective ear device for the oxygen tubing.

One CNL composed a team consisting of the nursing director, the CNLs, and staff nurses to use an interdisciplinary approach to find a solution to the problem. A product was identified, samples were requested, and a trial was completed with unsatisfactory results. The search continued for a prevention product. Finally, a soft silicone nasal cannula was found and trialed with improved outcomes. The number of stage 2 pressure ulcers decreased from 9 to 1 (89%) after the initiation of the soft nasal cannula on the medical unit.

A final example of a CNL's contribution to quality management occurred when the surgical unit staff at a hospital identified an increase in the incidence of pressure ulcers at the facility compared to the previous year. Working alongside the wound care nurse, a CNL reviewed education materials regarding pressure ulcers in patients with hip injuries and pressure ulcers in the sacral/buttocks areas gathered this information for the staff. The CNL's goal was to promote awareness and further education among the staff in the prevention of these wounds.

DISCUSSION QUESTIONS

1. Provide examples of how the CNL is held accountable for quality and safe outcomes.
2. What quality improvement initiatives related to patient issues can CNLs promote?

TEAM COORDINATION

The frontline team offers many suggestions and ideas for practice and environmental improvements during their shift. The CNL, acting as a liaison, can actively engage team members to help resolve the issue and/or implement an improvement strategy. For example, if a clinician has difficulty determining which vital signs are associated with the orthostatic blood pressures taken for her patient, the CNL can contact Information Services and describe what the clinician needs to see in the medical record. As a result, the appropriate view can be created. This would allow the clinician to treat the patient accordingly and in a more efficient manner.

Indwelling devices have the potential to cause infection the longer they are in place, which places patients at risk for adverse events, increased length of stay, and, ultimately, higher cost. A CNL's review includes the primary nurse and, at times, the physician to facilitate timely removal, thus lessening a chance for infection.

Transforming Care at the Bedside, or TCAB, is a national initiative sponsored by the Robert Wood Johnson Foundation and the Institute for Healthcare Improvement (IHI). The goal of TCAB is to address the quality of care on medical-surgical units and engage leaders at all levels of the organization while focusing on the work of one unit and ideas from frontline staff nurses.

One TCAB project created by a CNL at the author's hospital is a Welcome Binder and Welcome Bag for patients that are available upon arrival to the unit. The binders and bags are assembled by Central Supply; the bags belong to the patient and the binders are cleaned by housekeeping after a patient is discharged. The CNL's collaborative effort helped to enhance the patient experience. It also became a catalyst to engage staff in the process of changing work environments and improving patient outcomes.

The hospital has a monthly hospital-wide TCAB meeting with members from each nursing unit, Pharmacy, Dietary, Laboratory, and Central Supply. During these meetings, innovations are developed to "save time" for the staff nurses and improve working relationships with ancillary departments. As a result of the success on one medical unit, several other successful initiatives have been implemented hospital-wide. One success was a Central Line Kit that contains all the necessary items for a central line insertion so that staff do not have to hunt and gather in an emergency.

Staff also came up with the idea to place a sign on patient doors stating, "Do Not Disturb: Bedside Care in Progress." This helped to decrease interruptions and improve care rendered at the bedside. Another successful initiative was a "tape zone" around the medication dispensing machine Pyxis in an effort to decrease interruptions during medication administration. The tape zone was considered a best practice by The Joint Commission during its 2011 survey.

CNLs will continue to look for innovative ways to transform care at the bedside and to adapt new ideas to make lasting improvements in collaboration with ancillary departments. TCAB has been a great experience for all of the CNLs, nursing staff, patients, and the entire team at this author's hospital.

DISCUSSION QUESTIONS

1. How does the CNL include the frontline team in fostering quality initiatives?

2. How does the CNL and staff nurse relationship affect patient care outcomes?

3. What effect does the frontline team have on health care today?

RESOURCE ALLOCATION

Resource conservation is a way to curtail unit cost. Cost awareness of frequently used unit items by the staff raises awareness of capital expenditures. Readily accessible items encourage a less conservative approach to use. Environmental audits conducted by the CNLs help identify products that are duplicate or in excess use. Examples of this are often seen in isolation rooms because of gowning and gloving prior to each entry. Making essential resources available prevents the staff from "hunting and gathering" more items than needed.

Contaminated urine specimens increase cost, resulting in a delay of treatment, repetition of procedures, and duplication of processing. Education of the entire professional staff and patient care assistants is necessary to promote accurate specimen collection techniques. On one medical unit the rate of contaminated urine specimens was noted to be 47% (17/36). In collaboration with the Infection Prevention department, the unit's CNL developed an education program for the nursing staff to reinforce proper specimen collection techniques. After the education was completed, the unit observed an initial decrease in their contaminated urine specimens to 26% (10/39), then even lower, to 22% (13/54), over a 3-month period.

Another unit-specific CNL initiative that affected cost was creating a telemetry monitor sign-out/return book. This helped relocate and prevent the loss of telemetry monitors that cost $2,000 each. Prior to implementing this tracking system, three monitors were lost without any ability to trace their whereabouts, at a total cost of $6,000.

DISCUSSION QUESTIONS

1. Describe how the CNL employs cost reduction while not compromising the quality of health care.
2. How does the CNL serve as a responsible steward of the environment and human and material resources while coordinating care?
3. What unit-based initiatives reduced cost?

CARE MANAGEMENT

CNL student capstone projects can be implemented in practice settings. During one CNL student's role immersion, there was an increase in admissions on a unit due to warfarin-related issues. The CNL student identified this topic as an opportunity for staff and patient education.

The evidence-based literature demonstrates that knowledge of patients, families, and staff about warfarin prevents negative outcomes. Therefore, the student developed a warfarin education checklist for patients and nurses that was approved and implemented throughout the hospital. The checklist provided a systematic way of educating the staff and patients and acted as a visual reminder and resource. The goal was to reduce adverse outcomes and possible readmission of patients as a result of elevated prothrombin and International Normalized Ratios (INRs).

Qualitative outcomes are important to document. The patient/family experience during the hospital stay can affect the patient's recovery, outcomes, and prevention of adverse effects.

A high-quality patient experience will facilitate wellness and recovery. When a CNL's schedule is flexible, he or she can spend time with patients and families as needed. For example, a 40-year-old man was admitted to the intermediate care unit in heart failure. He had extensive cardiomyopathy and was a patient on the unit for 1 month. During his stay, the unit CNL met him daily in the "coffee shop" (the unit pantry). At the end of the month, the patient was transferred to another hospital for placement of a left ventricular access device (LVAC). He eventually received a heart transplant and called to tell the CNL about his heart transplant and to reiterate how those original meetings at the coffee shop helped him get through it all.

Two years later, the man still takes the opportunity to visit this CNL with a cup of coffee when he has his monthly blood work. The ongoing connection between CNL and patient resulted in a memorable positive experience for both parties.

DISCUSSION QUESTIONS

1. Describe how the CNL evaluates the environmental impact on health-care outcomes.

2. How does the CNL serve as the patient and family advocate in the acute care setting?

3. Describe how the CNL facilitates a positive patient–caregiver experience.

4. How does the CNL anticipate, plan for, and manage physical, psychological, social, and spiritual needs of the client and family or caregiver?

CLINICAL DECISION MAKING

CNLs have the opportunity to challenge current policy and procedures in clinical settings. With the emphasis on safe transitions to home after discharge from the hospital, postdischarge calls to patients have facilitated education, communication, prescription discussion, and follow-up appointments to prescribers. For example, a discharge call made to a patient after hip replacement surgery discovered that the patient was taking aspirin, 325 mg, every 4 hours instead of as ordered twice a day. The CNL consulted the patient's medical record to verify the actual dose the patient should have been taking with and alerted the physician that the patient had taken the extra doses. The CNL provided education to the patient regarding the appropriate frequency of the medication and then counseled the patient to follow up with the physician the next day.

Capturing the saves made by CNLs are essential data to collect in support of high-quality care, cost savings, and prevention of adverse postdischarge events.

DISCUSSION QUESTIONS

1. How does the CNL synthesize data, information, and knowledge on client outcomes and modify interventions to improve healthcare outcomes?

2. Describe how the CNL uses case management skills and principles in the delivery and supervision of client care across a continuum.

TRANSFORMATIONAL LEADERSHIP

CNLs are transformational leaders who seek new ways to achieve positive outcomes. They are vigilant in seeking innovative programs internally and externally that may enhance current practice. They support the implementation of projects, helping to direct where to start and who to include for each innovation. The CNL becomes the resource person because the ideas are intended to come from frontline staff members. Because change does not happen overnight, CNLs encourage the staff to try the innovation and remind them that they can adapt, adopt, or abandon the process if it fails. CNLs reinforce the idea that failure can be an acceptable outcome.

In one illustrative situation, a CNL identified the need to promote high-quality elder care in the acute care setting. The CNL accomplished this in collaboration with the director of the Office on Healthy Aging and director of Staff Development.

This author's organization selected the Nurses Improving Care for Healthsystem Elders (NICHE) evidence-based program to address the specialized needs of our elder population. NICHE was created in 1992 and is the only national geriatric nursing program encompassing more than 300 hospitals nationwide, as well as in Canada and the Netherlands. NICHE and the CNL role share quality indicators, such as prevention of falls, pressure ulcers, and infection and improvement of patient and nurse satisfaction. This similarity fostered combining the CNL/NICHE co-coordinator roles in our clinical setting.

The NICHE pilot program was initiated in an intermediate care unit that had a census of patients older than age 65. The CNLs on the unit developed and facilitated the NICHE volunteer program. The volunteers' goal is to enhance the patient experience by spending one-on-one time with patients, offering companionship and activities to support cognitive stimulation. The CNL offered Geriatric Resource Nurse (GRN) education to staff nurses who expressed an interest in further supporting the geriatric population. Six nurses completed the 20-hour e-learning program and received a certificate of completion. Their subsequent unit-based projects included offering advance directives, fostering mobility to prevent falls, and assessing and managing sleep, pain, oral hygiene, and sundowning/delirium. Because of the success of the pilot program, the NICHE program was then implemented on other units of the hospital with the ultimate goal of expanding to all other units (inpatient and outpatient) in the community.

DISCUSSION QUESTIONS

1. How is the CNL role transformational?
2. Innovation is paramount in health care. Identify ways the CNL has made a difference in the inpatient setting.
3. Describe the horizontal leadership role of the CNL on the healthcare team.

INFORMATICS

CNLs use information technology to retrieve current research and evidence-based practices to inform nursing practice. Understanding research methods and information technologies is necessary to effect positive patient outcomes. CNLs act as resource persons on the unit, using appropriate resources to find information. A CNL may also be the "superuser" of new equipment and help teach other nurses how to use healthcare equipment, as well as acting as a liaison between the Information Systems (IS) department and the staff. For example, when staff nurses identify a better way of communicating and documenting in the electronic medical record, the CNL can explain to the IS analyst the process that needs to be documented in a timely and efficient manner, and the analyst, with IT expertise, can input it into the system.

Some CNLs utilize skills in data management for TCAB interventions that are suggested by staff nurses. CNLs can also act as cheerleaders for projects, assisting in coordination of projects and supporting or mentoring staff nurses who devise with innovations. They build working relationships with interdisciplinary departments with a common goal of improving patient outcomes and giving time back to the bedside nurse.

DISCUSSION QUESTIONS

1. How does the CNL use information and communication technologies to document and evaluate client care, advance client education, and enhance the accessibility of care?

2. Describe how the CNL works on an interdisciplinary team to make ethical decisions regarding the application of technologies and the acquisition of data.

ILLNESS/DISEASE MANAGEMENT

Patients arrive in the acute care setting with a complex set of physical, psychological, and social challenges. Add that to a complex healthcare environment and it becomes challenging to meet their holistic needs. Syncope, for example, which is often accompanied by a fall at home, is a common admitting diagnosis in the acute care setting. Upon a patient's arrival to a unit, a CNL can assess the patient, identifying the safety risks while knowing that the patient needs to remain mobile to prevent deconditioning. The nurse obtains a set of orthostatic vital signs and then a prescriber's order of physical therapy is sought. The prescriber orders tests, and the CNL leads a discussion of this patient's case in staff rounds to evaluate whether the patient's medications contributed to the patient's syncope.

Depression is commonly seen among hospitalized patients as a result of prolonged illness and/or reduced capabilities. When, for example, a patient whose spouse has recently passed arrives on the unit, the CNL can contact the chaplain to come and offer support to the patient. The CNL may also order a consultation with Geriatrics to offer support measures to such a patient, such as counseling and medications. Such a patient often wants to return directly home but is advised by the healthcare team to spend a few days in a subacute rehabilitation facility to regain some strength in the lower extremities.

It is also common for elderly patients with arthritis to complain of continuous pain. The CNL can assist by discussing the issue with the patient, perhaps identifying that Tylenol (acetaminophen) was used at home with good effect. The CNL can then obtain an order for a standard dose of Tylenol to be given to the patient on a regular basis. As a result there is likely to be marked improvement in the patient's comfort and mobility during the rest of their hospital stay.

Conceptual Analysis of the CNL Role

The CNL is in a unique position to work alongside colleagues, witnessing the art and science of nursing at the bedside as the holistic needs of patients and their families are identified and addressed. Because the CNL is unit based, opportunities for coaching and mentoring staff to assume various roles in their career paths are readily available (Harris & Roussel, 2010).

The success of the CNL role results from support of the chief nursing officer (CNO), the chief executive officer (CEO), and each unit's nurse director. In these times of healthcare cost containment, the CNO and CEO must justify the financial expenditure of hiring CNLs within their organization. The leadership of people in these positions enables CNLs to be innovative, ground breaking, and pioneers of the role. Monthly meetings with the CNO and nurse directors enable a discussion of unit-based initiatives, upcoming presentations, and future goals.

CNLs from the author's organization have attended national CNL conferences and presented posters on the previously mentioned falls prevention and facilitation of the NICHE program. One publication by the CNLs at our organization include "CNLs Make a Difference!" in *Nursing* (Sheets et al., 2012). These presentations and publications reflect the CNL's role and initiatives.

Currently, one CNL in the author's organization is a member of the CNL Expert Panel for the American Association of Colleges of Nursing. One of the charges of this panel was to evaluate and update the white paper on the education and role of the clinical nurse leader (AACN, 2007) and to review the CNL exam.

The development of the CNL role at our organization has been a fluid process, with few to no restrictions set by leadership as to what the role should be. CNL leadership is fostered such that the boundaries of the role are not defined so much as guided by *White Paper on the Education and Role of the Clinical Nurse Leader* (AACN, 2007) and the role is allowed to develop and grow. With administration's support, the CNLs have a strong foundation at this hospital and will continue to expand their innovations in an effort to improve safety and patient outcomes.

References

American Association of Colleges of Nursing. (2007). *White paper on the education and role of the Clinical Nurse Leader.* Retrieved from http://www.nursing.vanderbilt.edu/msn/pdf/cm_AACN_CNL.pdf

Harris, J. L., & Roussel, L. A. (2010). *Initiating and sustaining the clinical nurse leader role: A practical guide.* Sudbury, MA: Jones and Bartlett Publishers.

Inouye, S. K., Brown, C. J., & Tinetti, M. E. (2009). Medicare nonpayment, hospital falls, and unintended consequences. *New England Journal of Medicine, 360,* 2390–2393. Retrieved from http://www.nejm.org/doi/full/10.1056/NEJMp0900963

Institute of Medicine. (2011). *The future of nursing: Leading change, advancing health.* Washington, DC: National Academies Press.

Office of Nursing Services. (2009). *VA nursing: Connecting all the pieces to transform care for the veterans.* Retrieved from http://www.va.gov/NURSING/docs/OfficeofNursingServices-ONS_Annual_Report_2009-WEB.pdf

Sheets, M., Bonnah, B., Kareivis, J., Abraham, P., Sweeney, M., & Strauss, J. (2012). CNLs make a difference! *Nursing, 42*(8), 54–58.

Tornabeni, J. (2006). The evolution of a revolution in nursing. *Journal of Nursing Administration, 36*(1), 3–6.

CHAPTER **13**

Disaster Preparedness

Dottie Bringle, RN, BSN, MSHSA, COO/CNO, Mercy-Joplin Hospital

Learning Objectives

At the completion of this chapter, you will be able to:

1. Identify culturally responsive strategies for disaster preparedness.
2. Increase master's-prepared nurses' awareness of their roles and responsibilities in disaster preparedness.
3. Evaluate effective responses to disaster efforts across the life span.
4. Identify community supports during the recovery phase of a disaster.
5. Outline effective planning strategies necessary for disaster preparedness in the workplace and community.

Part I: Joplin, Missouri

Joplin, Missouri, is a community of approximately 50,000 people. It is located in the southwest corner of the state. We are surrounded by several rural communities in the four-state region. Our population actually surges (i.e., doubles) during the week and weekends as a result of people commuting to Joplin to work and shop. There are two hospitals in Joplin, St. John's Regional Medical Center and Freeman Hospital. Both tertiary referral hospitals are of similar size and capability as Level II trauma centers.

Part II: Disaster Management

St. John's has always been very involved in disaster management. Every year it performs several drills, and participation in these drills is not optional. When a drill is called, it is expected that protocols for that specific disaster are implemented. All areas of the hospital have access to the disaster plan both electronically and in hard copy format. Administrators are also expected to participate; incident command is established immediately and management is expected to move into the areas of the hospital to ensure staff are participating. St. John's had, in 2011, actually participated in and coordinated efforts with the city of Joplin, Jasper County, the Emergency Healthcare Coalition, Region D, and the state of Missouri. Even though our plan was considered to be comprehensive, it did not go far enough because we never planned for total destruction.

Part III: May 22, 2011: Joplin Tornado

On May 22, 2011, at 5:41 p.m. our 367-bed facility, St. John's Regional Medical Center (now named Mercy Hospital–Joplin), took a direct hit by a devastating EF5 tornado (a tornado of the most devastating level). Wind gusts of up to 250 miles per hour hit our community. The tornado's path was 13.8 miles long, and it created a 1-mile-wide band of complete destruction. As the tornado was tracked across our community, it was believed that the EF5 tornado formed and made its first direct hit on St. John's. As Diane Sawyer of ABC News so eloquently spoke:

> There was silence and then the roar was like that of a freight train. The sound was deafening and the pressure was unbelievable; 45 seconds later and it was over. The tornado hit the

west side of the building, filled the infrastructure and blew out all the windows and walls, as well as portions of the roof were pulled off. Much of the building's infrastructure was severely damaged or destroyed. (ABC News, 2011)

A few short seconds changed the lives of many in our community. This event is not something any of us will ever forget.

"We are in a dire situation" was the message from the PBX operator (on the private branch exchange) before the line went dead. In southwest Missouri, it is not unusual to have severe weather in spring and early summer. This particular day, many have since stated, people felt was "somehow different" and therefore took the severe weather warnings more seriously. This feeling likely saved many lives. Tammy Fritchey, an intensive care unit registered nurse, said some didn't immediately start following "condition grey" protocols. She said she told them, "No, we are going to do this the correct way. Something feels different today." Thankfully, the staff did follow the emergency protocols that we had drilled many times in the past.

There were 183 inpatients and 25 emergency department (ED) patients in the building at the time the tornado struck. Parts of the hospital were still standing but not safe. After digging themselves out of the rubble, the hospital staff had no idea the entire hospital was mortally wounded. What they knew was that whichever area they were in was not safe. The hospital was filling with the odor of natural gas from a ruptured gas line. The ceiling tiles were falling down, doors had been blown off their hinges, water was standing in the hallways, emergency lighting had been pulled from the walls, and the building was very dark. Cell phones and flashlights became the only sources of light.

Doctors and nurses put in chest tubes, intubated patients, and bandaged gaping wounds amid the destruction. They instructed families on how to care for their loved ones until they could get them to Freeman Hospital. Yet, because it was the only building that remained standing for many blocks around, people from the community flooded into the hospital. Many people were bleeding and crying. One unit clerk, who had worked at St. John's only a few weeks, described a young mother who ran through the door holding a baby covered in blood. The mother threw the baby into the clerk's arms and asked her if her baby was dead.

Evacuation was the only thing to do. The staff immediately began doing what they were trained to do, and in 90 minutes they had the entire hospital evacuated. Patients were staged by the stairwells of their respective units and prepared to evacuate the building. Dennis Manley, director of Risk and Quality Management, described that there were three different collection points outside of the building because there was no single way out of the destruction from within the hospital. Staff cared for patients in the parking lots, amid all the twisted metal of vehicles, our BK-117 helicopter, and a sea of disoriented people and small animals. Many continued to go back into the building to get patients out, even when the fire department said there was smoke coming from the building. Ensuring the safety of their patients, even above their own well-being, was paramount. As it turned out, the building was not on fire and the smoke was actually from oxygen tanks that had erupted and were spewing oxygen into the atmosphere. Many believe that if the generators had not been destroyed, the hospital indeed would have caught on fire, and probably many would have been electrocuted.

Many heroes came into being on this horrible day. Ambulatory patients walked. Other patients were carried on backboards, doors, mattresses, and other evacuation devices down the stairwells of the nine-story building. Critical patients were loaded into pickup trucks and other private vehicles to be transported to our competitor hospital, Freeman, which was about 6 blocks away. The less critical patients were taken to our rehabilitation hospital, which was severely damaged but was the only building on our 50-acre-plus campus that was not totally destroyed and had limited generator power.

Manley described approaching the hospital in total disbelief. He saw destroyed homes, cars twisted into unrecognizable shapes, downed power lines, and massive piles of debris littering the streets and grounds. Trees resembled stick figures because the bark had been blown off. The area looked like a war zone. Many were overheard saying they had never seen destruction of this magnitude, even in wartime. Many had considered the hospital indestructible, with its generators and redundant systems that would bring it through any storm. Unfortunately, this time it would not survive the wrath of Mother Nature.

Staff were forced to practice wartime medicine and saw death and destruction they will never forget. Once patients were evacuated and sent to area hospitals, the staff began to walk to Memorial Hall, previously a concert venue, where they set up triage and treatment areas for the community. They carried armloads of supplies and pushed wheelchairs with supplies and equipment loaded in them to the Hall, nearly 3 miles from the hospital. McAuley High School gymnasium also became a refuge for people who had no homes left and who simply needed shelter and a place for minor treatment and comfort.

Communication was our biggest dilemma. Telephone lines were down and radio lines were for emergency traffic only. If not for texting, it would have been nearly impossible for caregivers to communicate with each other.

It has been estimated that nearly 1,500 people were treated in the first 24 hours. Because we were on generator power, triage had to become very focused and X-rays were done only if a patient's life was threatened. Typical injuries were degloving injuries, people impaled by objects, lacerations, and broken bones. Pain medications and oxygen were extremely limited. Many people who arrived from private homes and nursing homes required oxygen, and there was virtually none available (the local vendor for oxygen tanks was also destroyed). E-cylinders were located and steps were taken to "make do" until alternatives could be located. Mercy Health System, St. John's parent company, owns our supply chain vendor, ROi. ROi immediately went into action to provide supplies. Their trucks, 75 miles away, were loaded with supplies and medications they thought would be most needed and were immediately sent to Joplin. What an absolute blessing this was, as staff tirelessly provided care for our community.

The next day, as the emergency operation began to settle down somewhat, it became important to move our command center away from Memorial Hall. We moved to a local trade center and had to immediately move from emergency mode to our next step of disaster management: recovery. Lynn Britton,

Mercy's chief executive officer, and Mike McCurry, Mercy's chief operating officer, came to Joplin with other team members to help our local team sort out our next steps. They provided support and resources, but never did they "take over" local operation.

Our building had been destroyed; however, to quote Sue Hall, an emergency department RN, "St. John's the building is gone. St. John's the heart ... we just moved."

Missouri Disaster Medical Assistance Team (DMAT) came to the command center and told us of a field hospital, a mobile medical unit, they had set up for training in Branson, Missouri. They suggested it might provide us with an alternate hospital in which to continue to provide care for our community. On Tuesday, May 24, 2011, we went to Branson to look at what would become our next hospital. With the help of the Missouri National Guard and the Missouri DMAT, by 1 a.m. on Thursday morning our field hospital was set up and ready to begin service. This small facility gave our hospital community a boost of energy and hope. We were, in fact, rebuilding and beginning to heal.

On Sunday morning, May 29, at 7:00 a.m., exactly one week after our hospital was destroyed, we were ready to see our first patient, who arrived at 7:03. The excitement was clearly visible on every face at our new hospital. Important to note: We not only had staff, equipment, and supplies to continue our mission to care for our community but also fully electronic medical records and new Omnicell drug cabinets in place and functioning. The field hospital had 60 beds; a pharmacy; mobile CT, MRI, and X-ray; a nuclear lab; two self-contained operating rooms; a mobile catheter lab; a laboratory; a dietary area; and security. We treated about 100 patients per day in our ED and kept approximately 25 inpatients per day. We ran on generator power for several weeks and were forced to utilize portable restrooms and bedside commodes. We did have running water, although it was limited. With the field hospital, we knew we had only met a temporary need and would have to move quickly to secure our next-phase facility.

About 10 days after the disaster, we were visited by U.S. Air Force Surgeon General (Ret.) P. K. Carlton. He had spent his career managing disasters in the United States and overseas. He let us know very quickly that we could not be satisfied with the field hospital and offered suggestions to help us move forward. He talked about other tragedies in U.S. history and abroad. Immediately, we made plans to travel to California to visit with individuals who had worked with General Carlton and to discuss options for our next phases.

It was determined we would utilize a modular-type facility that would allow for actual patient rooms with windows, doors, running water, and flushing toilets. The facility plan was laid out on the same basic footprint as the field hospital. Careful steps were taken to ensure that as we took down sections of the field hospital they were replaced with the modular units. Embedded into the overall floor plan, this facility had 10 ICU beds, 36 medical-surgical beds, and all the other services of the field hospital. While the modular facility was being constructed, we determined we would need to bring in modular clinic facilities because many of our medical staff had no offices to work from. We completely moved in to the modular facility on October 2, 2011. In this same period of time, a 32-bed Behavioral Health inpatient unit was opened as well as facilities for outpatient behavioral health services.

All the time we were planning and building the modular facility we also were completing plans for the third and final phases of our recovery to normal operations. On April 15, 2012, a component hospital was completed just to the south of the modular facility. This hospital would be the permanent facility until the new replacement hospital opens in the spring of 2015. The component hospital is 150,000 square feet. It has state-of-the-art facilities: four large surgery suites; two catheter labs; an electrophysiology (EP) lab; a 27-bed emergency department; and an inpatient bed capacity of 110 beds, which includes our labor/delivery/recovery/postpartum (LDRP) and pediatric units. We were able to once again perform open-heart procedures.

The new replacement hospital is located about 3 miles south of Joplin where Main Street and I-44 intersect. The groundbreaking took place on January 29, 2012, with plans for a spring 2015 opening. Mercy will rebuild this new hospital with 327 inpatient beds to support the region, and it will have expansion capacity for up to 424 beds. The new footprint will allow Mercy to deliver health care in a new way. It will be built with the patients' comfort and ease of use in mind. This facility will also offer a neonatal intensive care unit (NICU), which the destroyed hospital did not have.

Part IV: Mercy's Commitment

Mercy remained committed to the Joplin employees throughout the disaster and recovery. When Mercy's top leadership heard of the destruction of its hospital in Joplin, they immediately began the process of taking care of employees. Lynn Britton, Mercy's CEO, immediately announced that all 2,200 coworkers would continue to receive their pay checks and everything would be done to keep them with "meaningful work." Overnight, Mercy Health System created the largest employment agency in the state of Missouri—a process that was later called Talent Share. The organization worked with other organizations and the employees to send employees to hospitals and agencies in the surrounding areas that needed their particular expertise. The employees continued to receive their normal pay and benefits, as well as mileage and expenses if they had to leave the immediate area. Also, a relief fund was set up to assist employees who had personally suffered losses of their homes, cars, and personal effects. In August 2012, several employees were still in Talent Share roles and will likely remain so until the opening of the new replacement hospital in 2015.

Mercy's commitment to the community is unwavering. By the time the new hospital is built, Mercy will have reinvested approximately $958 million into our community. This is true commitment. "Our ministry has never been confined to a building. Our people and our spirit are at the core of who we are and what we do. We are rising from the rubble stronger than ever before," said Britton.

Part V: Realistic Labor Allocation

When disaster strikes it can be fast, furious, without forewarning, and crippling. The type of disaster and extent of destruction determine your most immediate needs. In our case, when the weather station began releasing footage, which was almost immediately, volunteers in areas of the community not affected began to show up. *Do not underestimate the human resources requirements and do not underestimate the value of volunteers.* If you do not assign people to a task, they will search for ways to assist on their own.

During the first few hours, through the next day, and over the next week, our human resources issues included the following:

- Triage sites were set up in three different locations outside of the hospital, east drive/parking, north parking lot/street, and south side of the hospital.
- Staff and volunteers worked to evacuate our hospital in 90 minutes by working together. Critical care staff stayed with their patients during transport and as they reached their respective locations to assist in provision of care.
- Volunteers who were able to get close to the hospital in their pickups and SUVs were recruited to transport patients. More than 350 people were transported in the first hour after the storm.
- Runners and people to communicate are essential if you have no working communication devices.
- Supply coordinator.
- Supply vendor (ROi).
- Pharmacists to manage drug inventory.
- Logistics persons to identify where patients are transferred.
- Security to secure the site as soon as possible.
- Search and rescue teams.
- Public relations coordinator as the point of contact for agencies.

Once the decision was made to relocate to an alternate site, human resources issues included these:

- Physicians, nurses, and ancillary clinicians as well as other staff to provide care at Memorial Hall
- Operations, planning, and logistics persons to set up treatment sites and create some semblance of order
- Staffing coordinators to manage staffing requirements

- Medical records and IT to ensure stability of records and computer system (Joplin went live with our electronic health records on May 1, 2011.)
- Persons to contact families of deceased as well as manage flow of patients, that is, where patients were transferred
- Supply and equipment coordinator

After the first 24 to 48 hours, other human resources needs became critical. Examples of these are as follows:

- Food services for staff and workers
- Facilities coordination (lighting, security, and/or National Guard to secure site and buildings; personnel to take care of generator needs, hand washing stations, portable toilets, transportation vehicles, tents for meetings/gatherings, shower and laundry facilities; persons to identify owners of vehicles, enable people to retrieve their personal vehicles, and interact with private insurance companies; people to manage site preparation and construction needs)
- Supply chain to secure needed equipment and supplies for immediate patient care as well as for new field hospital
- Warehousing
- Badging, credentialing, and tracking
- Biomedical technicians to ensure equipment is safe for use
- Persons to interface with government and regulatory agencies
- Volunteer coordinator (Volunteers from outside of your community will come in large numbers.)
- Coordinator to manage donations both internally and to other locations throughout the city
- Counselors and social workers
- Persons to work with vendors and negotiate costs for equipment and other needs (We recommend this person be away from the site but connected to the person in charge at the site.)
- Representative at the local Emergency Planning agency to act as a liaison (Communication initially with governing agencies is critical.)

- Incident command (This should be set up away from the disaster site.) and the following people:
  - Finance
  - Clinical
  - Infection control
  - Secretarial support
  - Logistics
  - Public relations
  - Human resources
  - Information technology
  - PBX operators (We received 2,500 calls within first 24 hours.)
  - Persons to attend Federal Emergency Management Administration (FEMA) and city/state meetings to ensure your organization is well represented

Resource needs can be overwhelming and extensive. St. John's was fortunate to have become part of the Mercy Health System in November 2009. As a result, we had access to many resources from across our system.

DISCUSSION QUESTIONS

1. What risks did Mercy–St. John's identify predisaster and how did they plan to mitigate those risks?
2. What activities were put in place to reduce loss of life and property predisaster?
3. How did Mercy–St. John's safeguard the community during the disaster?
4. What role or roles for the general public did Mercy–St. John's identify to mitigate risk?

Part VI: Interacting with the Agencies: Pre/During/Post Disaster

As previously stated, Mercy–St. John's had always been very involved in disaster preparedness. Drills were held several times per year. Even in the middle of our rebuilding efforts, the importance of being ready continued to be a focus. The motto "Drill until you fail, then drill again" is utilized. There is absolutely no substitute for the drills you do. Decisions must be made at the lowest levels. The fact that everyone was so well trained speaks to why more people were not hurt or killed in the disaster and why so many were able to reach safety quickly. It is imperative that staff go through the drills and know their emergency procedures so they can act intuitively in the time of a disaster—large or small and with or without their emergency manual/protocols to assist them.

Being part of Mercy Health System gave us access to resources from across the ministry. Expertise could be pulled from other organizations as could vendors, who stood ready to assist with some of our plant issues, such as securing the building, retrieving items from the building, and renovating buildings that had minimal damage. If you do not have a large health system to back you up, you clearly need to understand what your resources are from local, state, and federal perspectives.

Following are examples of local, state, and federal resources:

- *City management (Department of Health/city manager/ emergency coordinator):* Know the people you will be working with in your local and city government. Have their contact information in your computer as well as on your cell phone.
- *Missouri DMAT:* Identify the commander as well as the chief medical officer. They were of great value in moving forward and offered "pearls of wisdom" on how to interact with other agencies.
- *National Guard:* The Guard assisted in the construction of the field hospital. They also provided great assistance in securing property and curbing vandalism.
- *Missouri Hospital Association/Mo-DHHS/Governor's Office:* Utilize your state hospital association to assist with needed resources, whether equipment, staff, or processing. It is of great help in obtaining waivers and provision of resources to identify areas of needed assistance.
- *Governor's Office:* Our Governor's Office sent resources to our community to identify specific needs where the governor could help. The governor spent considerable time in

our community helping the hospital, school district, and others in removing barriers.

- *SEMA/FEMA:* It is important to immediately connect with the State Emergency Management Agency (SEMA) and FEMA representative who is assigned to your facility. If you are unfamiliar with the Robert T. Stafford Disaster Relief and Emergency Assistance Act, it is important for someone to have access to it. Recommend hiring an agency to assist with coordination of FEMA process. Following the FEMA guidelines carefully places your organization at less risk of losing any potential funding.
- *FEMA Environmental and Historic Preservation:* As repair and rebuilding take place in communities, environmental and historic preservation concerns may seem unimportant. Do not fall into the trap of ignoring or minimizing the importance of these laws. Failure to comply with applicable environmental and historic laws could jeopardize or delay any potential funding.
- *U.S. Army Corps of Engineers:* Discussions with the Corps took place almost immediately. They will work hand in hand with FEMA, and meetings are smoother and quicker when both of these agencies are in the same room at the same time.
- *Law enforcement:* Local law enforcement played a significant role in assisting to secure our buildings and premises. Many agencies were deployed to our community.
- *Federal agencies:* The Department of Health and Human Services; Homeland Security; local, state, and federal legislators as well as the president of the United States came to Joplin. It is important to have a delegation of people available who can assist in telling your story and communicating your specific needs. When people offer a card or contact information, in case they can help, take this information readily. You will likely need it at a later date.
- *Joint Commission/Centers for Medicare and Medicaid Services:* Both agencies came to visit our temporary facilities. They were helpful and offered good advice to help ensure safety measures were in place.

DISCUSSION QUESTIONS

1. How did Mercy–St. John's provide public education and evaluate their emergency preparedness in advance to prepare for evacuation?

2. What changes, if any, would you recommend for Mercy–St. John's in their disaster preparedness plan?

3. Did Mercy–St. John's have an adequately prepared nursing workforce to respond to this disaster? Why or why not?

4. What policies related to the use of unlicensed personnel from outside of the disaster jurisdiction would you create?

5. What types of community needs assessments can nurses do to prepare for a disaster?

6. What role can nurses play in activities such as equipment and supply needs, training, shelter, and communication during disasters such as this?

It is important to continue to communicate and interact with these agencies on an ongoing basis. Conversations should occur with specified individuals to ensure continuity and consistency in messaging as well as to ensure all necessary steps are taking place as you move forward. Do not take for granted the resources that are available. It is better to prepare in advance than to wait until there is an actual disaster.

- Does your disaster management plan go far enough?
- Does your facility "drill until you fail"?
- If your facility lost all redundant backup systems and it came down only to staff knowledge of how to handle the disaster, would staff know what to do?
- Are you *ready*?

DISCUSSION QUESTIONS

1. How would you determine whether standards of care need to be altered during a disaster?

2. Do you feel prepared to provide care in a variety of settings under challenging conditions? If not, how will you prepare?

3. What is the community's responsibility to individuals with chronic disease or disability during a disaster?

4. How would you use your skills in epidemiology to identify and plan for health hazards during a disaster?

5. What, if any, additional services may be needed at an institution like Mercy–St. John's as they recover and rebuild their healthcare infrastructure?

6. Develop three to five outcome criteria that you would use to evaluate a disaster plan.

Reference

ABC News. (2011, May 24). Joplin tornado: Doctors rush to save lives. Diane Sawyer reports. Retrieved from http://abcnews.go.com/GMA/video/joplin-tornado-doctors-saving-lives-13672515

© Leksusluss/ShutterStock, Inc.

CHAPTER **14**

Power in the Healthcare Relationship

Judith B. Krauss, RN, MSN, FAAN

Learning Objectives

At the completion of this chapter, you will be able to:

1. Discuss organizational management: basic elements of group process and structure, aspects of intergroup relationships, organizational culture, values, and work behavior.
2. Discuss effective group leadership and membership: authority, power, change.
3. Develop an awareness of how power is used in the healthcare relationship.
4. Discuss the use and abuse of power in the healthcare relationship.
5. Discuss competencies and essential qualities for effective leadership.

Background

The healthcare relationship is contextual. It spans the interpersonal level, which focuses on patient–clinician interaction, and

299

the systems level, which includes organizational and policy factors. Patients and practitioners have health encounters that may constitute the basis for a relationship over time, may be time limited by the duration of a specific illness, or may be one-time occurrences. Although patient–practitioner interactions involve a complex set of variables, an important and little examined variable is the power dynamic that exists in virtually every healthcare exchange. According to Hill (1995), power can be defined as the

> potential of an individual (or group) to influence another individual or group. Influence, in turn, is the exercise of power to change the behavior, attitudes, and/or values of that individual or group. It is easier to change behavior than attitudes, and in turn, attitudes than values. (p. 24)

The last decades have challenged the traditional medical model of the healthcare relationship in which physicians were accorded ultimate power and authority over healthcare decisions based on their years of education, special scientific knowledge, and sheer social stature. Influences such as the growth of technology and greater availability of healthcare information to the lay public (Cassell, 1991); greater emphasis on individual and organizational empowerment (Freire, 1972; Grossman & Valiga, 2005; Tomey, 2000); increased diversity of the population; proliferation of healthcare practitioner roles, including the more independent roles of nurse practitioners and physician assistants; and the introduction of managed care have all contributed to a complex healthcare paradigm and changed the power relations between and among practitioners, patients, and healthcare organizations. Today, the healthcare relationship is variously described using terms such as *mutuality, partnership, respect, autonomy,* and *shared decision making.* All of these terms are about power, who has it, and how it is shared in the context of the healthcare relationship.

Healthcare professionals derive power from education, licensure, social status, and the personal intimacy they are afforded in healthcare encounters. Power affects actual and perceived rewards, accountability, and responsibility, as well as interprofessional and patient–practitioner relationships. The power balance between a nurse and patient is different from that between doctor and patient and different yet from that between X-ray technician and patient. However, healthcare professionals are reluctant to acknowledge the language of power when describing clinical transactions with patients and others. For those in the helping professions, the relationship with the patient is often a more powerful influence on healing and recovery than expert knowledge per se (Cassell, 1991). Yet, power within and among the health professions is often based on expert rather than relational knowledge.

For years issues related to the balance of power in the healthcare relationship have captured the attention of medical ethicists. However, ethical perspectives on the power dynamic between patients and practitioners have also changed with time. Where there once was an almost exclusive focus on the philosophic concerns of rights and principles of freedom, self-determination, and autonomy, there is now a focus on clinical pragmatism, the tensions between a rights ethic and a care ethic, the moral problems presented by the healthcare relationship itself, the notion of obligations that accompany rights, and an examination of autonomy in these contexts (Alcabes & Williams, 2002; Fins, 1999; Fins, Miller, & Bacchetta, 1998; Fins & Solomon, 2001; Henderson & Fins, 1998; Levi, 1999; Yoder, 2002). The intersection of bioethics and the healthcare relationship, particularly as relates to the balance of power between patient and practitioner, deserves greater attention not only in health professions education but also in the day-to-day practice arena where these issues unfold. Yet, we have little useful information about these day-to-day exchanges.

One way of accessing the power perspective of day-to-day patient–practitioner interactions is through the personal narrative. The personal narrative allows an individual to tell a whole story from a particular perspective. This chapter offers a collection of "power stories" told by graduate nursing students. Excerpts from the stories represented here have been harvested from approximately 130 final-year students enrolled in a graduate nursing program. Stories were collected over two academic years as part of the course assignment in a course that emphasized the importance of context in understanding policy formation as well as individual and organizational dynamics. Students were informed that the stories would be used in a published chapter and were asked to use pseudonyms and otherwise disguise the identities of people and places involved. They were given an early draft of this chapter and offered the option of withdrawing their stories from consideration—none were withdrawn.

The student assignment was to write a vignette concerning power—either representing power dynamics at the level of the nurse–patient transaction or at the organizational or systems level (for example, between clinicians, between a clinician and administrator, between the healthcare organization and an outside agent such as a regulator or insurer). Students were asked to describe incidents they had observed firsthand about which they had detailed knowledge and information. The story could be about the appropriate or inappropriate use of power from the student's perspective. Students were asked to provide detailed accounts such that the reader could vicariously live the incident through the student's narrative and to provide a written assessment of the power dynamics using the following guidelines:

- Identify the relevant parties and the interdependencies among them. Who is dependent on whom and for what? Whose cooperation is needed? Whose compliance?
- Determine the sources of power of the relevant parties (e.g., positional, personal, or both).
- Determine the similarities and differences among the parties in terms of goals, values, stake in the outcome, and/or working styles. What are the underlying factors that create differences in these areas (e.g., information, education, position in the organization, socioeconomic background, career plans)?
- Identify the broader context? How much potential for conflict exists? Are there precipitating factors? Is the organization undergoing major change?
- Determine what led to the conclusion that the incident represents an appropriate or inappropriate use of power.

Stories selected for the chapter were those that illustrated themes oft repeated in many of the submissions and, as a collection, illustrated the full range of stories submitted. The stories are colored by the narrators' roles as students, their relationships with faculty and preceptors, the existing power dynamics between nurses and doctors, and the ever present interpersonal and organizational dynamics that are embedded in all healthcare relationships. Taken together they constitute a unique and valuable collection that begins to capture the role of power in the healthcare relationship through a nursing lens—notable for the emphasis on the misuse of power even though the assignment invited stories that illustrated the appropriate as well as inappropriate use of power.

The stories fall naturally into four relational categories:

- Nurse–patient relationships
- Interprofessional relationships
- Student–faculty relationships
- Systems relationships

Nurse–Patient Relationships

Within this category there were three different types of stories. A number of stories emphasized the theme of the patient's or family's power over health professionals and the treatment plan. Another group of stories highlighted the theme of the practitioner's positive or negative use of power in the patient–practitioner interaction. And a third focused on the healthcare professional as patient or family member.

Patients and families can knowingly or unknowingly influence healthcare transactions. There is an aspect of the patient–practitioner transaction, particularly in hospitals and clinics, that is quite public and poses the powerful threat of embarrassment or humiliation or even threatens the safety of the nurse. Sometimes just the anticipation of such events is enough to influence the behavior of the nurse or other healthcare professionals in the clinical situation. Families also have a powerful influence on healthcare transactions. They can be an important source of information or a barrier to information. They can positively or negatively affect the patient's cooperation with treatment. In the case of children, elders, or adults with disabling conditions, the nurse must attend to family dynamics.

Similarly, certain interactions between health professionals and patients are more easily observed and highlight the power dynamic. Finally, nurses who themselves have been patients or who have been involved as the family member of a patient have a unique perspective on the power dynamic in the healthcare relationship.

CASE STUDIES

THE POWER OF PATIENTS AND FAMILIES

CASE 1: Mr. R.

Mr. R. was 2 days post-op after an insertion of a baclofen pump into his spinal column to help manage muscle spasms secondary to multiple sclerosis (MS). During surgery a nerve was irritated, causing pain 9/10 down his right leg. Pain from the multiple incisional sites was well controlled at 1/10. According to Mr. R, the MDs managing the case were aware of his pain management problems and the day shift nurse had told him that the acute pain service would stop by to speak with him. In fact the pain service had already signed off his case. I had not received report from the day nurse (she had gone home) and there was no documentation of Mr. R's pain management plan of care. Mr. R. also told me that he was receiving a lesser dose of Neurontin (gabapentin) than what he took at home. He wanted me to contact his primary neurologist so that the neurologist could become involved in his plan of care, especially pain management. The resident in pain management insisted that he could not increase the Neurontin dose and he was unable to add additional interventions to control Mr. R's pain. He further expressed his irritation about the involvement of the primary neurologist. . . . Mr. R had upset the power balance by adding his outpatient neurologist to the mix.

CASE 2: Mr. F.

Mr. F is a 42-year-old man with a history of heroin abuse. He presented for follow-up of a lower-respiratory infection and new onset fatigue. He complained of insomnia and requested some of the painkillers he had received for a prior episode of back pain. Although he was enrolled in the Methadone treatment program he had not been to clinic in several weeks and admitted to recently using heroin. He declined attempts to reestablish care at the Methadone clinic, saying that he couldn't afford the services. When I suggested that his insomnia might be a side effect of either methadone withdrawal or heroin use and that pain meds would just be a "Band-Aid" solution to the real problem, he became very agitated and verbally combative. Feeling threatened and unsure of the situation, I said I needed to consult my preceptor. He agreed, aware that I was a student. My preceptor returned with me to the exam room where Mr. F gave her the same history but added the complaint of back pain. Despite various attempts on the part of the preceptor to address the situation and nearly 10 minutes of reasoning and offers to help Mr. F, he began calling her a wimp: "You're just a wimp. Help me out here." In the end, we sought the help of Dr. W, a tall, fairly robust physician who emphasized to Mr. F that he had an addiction that required treatment. Mr. F left the office empty-handed.

CASE 3: THE ED

While working in the ED, I was assigned a hallway. Typically, patients in the hallway are those who don't need critical care, psychiatric patients awaiting medical clearance to go to the psychiatric unit, and intoxicated individuals. I had an intoxicated man who was rather obnoxious. When he was brought in he was not restrained (though that is the usual practice for people who are intoxicated). He was harassing females, asking if he could grab their breast and buttocks and making other inappropriate verbal expressions. I had been given verbal orders to medicate him with Haldol (haloperidol) to help him get to sleep.

I had just gotten him to agree to the shot when the daughter of one of the other patients approached to ask whether I needed help (she actually worked as a tech in our ED). Unfortunately, this set the man off again and he began his verbal abuse anew. At this point, a male tech came over to assist despite my request that he let me handle the situation. He grabbed the man's arm, attempting to restrain him.

Soon thereafter we had the male charge nurse involved, and a female resident, witnessing the commotion, decided to call security. It was not long before two security guards and one other random person were also at the bedside. By this time I had been pushed out of the way. The man ended up in four-point restraints. The charge nurse had put a sheet over the man's face because the man had reverted to spitting. I eventually was able to give him the Haldol and within 5 minutes he was asleep.

CASE 4: Mr. J.

Mr. J is a 69-year-old man with dementia, mental retardation, and uncontrolled hypertension whose health visits are directed by a domineering niece who treats him poorly and seldom lets him speak for himself. According to the chart note from his last visit, once his niece left the room Mr. J was able to articulate surprisingly well and stated that when his niece is around "it's just easier to sit there and shut up." As I began my interview with Mr. J, his niece informed me, "He doesn't understand you, he's stupid—he has the mind of a five-year-old." The niece and her mother (Mr. J's sister) had recently learned that Mr. J had stopped taking his blood pressure medication. On physical exam he had a blood pressure of 220/110 mm Hg and remarkable swelling of his left lower extremity. We decided to send Mr. J to the ER to get his blood pressure under control and to rule out a deep-vein thrombosis. Visibly annoyed, the niece said, "I knew this was going to happen!" We decided to send Mr. J to the ER via ambulance because we could not rely on the family to manage this through outpatient visits.

CASE 5: Mrs. X

Sarah's mom (Mrs. X) was having difficulty with the way the surgical team was managing her daughter's care. But instead of talking to them about it or requesting to speak to the nurse manager or one of the house officers, she reacted by yelling and crying. It was during one of these emotional outbursts that I first met Mrs. X. I passed by as she was speaking heatedly with the surgical team in the hallway. Within a matter of seconds, the conversation escalated with mom yelling loudly, crying, and swearing while I and four other nurses sat wide-eyed in the conference room....

The next evening I discovered that Sarah had been assigned as one of my patients. I was dreading the assignment, feeling relatively new and inexperienced, and not looking forward to the possibility that Mrs. X would take issue with my care.... I had been intimidated by parents before but never actually felt scared of one until now....

The night was going relatively well until about 10 p.m. when Mrs. X called me into the room, concerned that Sarah had been sleeping on the chest tube and it was slightly crimped. Sarah was crying slightly. Mrs. X was very upset but did not want me to assess the situation and did not want my input. She demanded I call pain service immediately, which I did. The resident came within minutes of my call and went to see Sarah. It did not appear to him that Sarah was in pain, but to appease Mrs. X he ordered an X-ray and increased Sarah's pain medication even though it didn't seem necessary.

CASE 6: THE PICU

A 3-year-old boy was admitted to the PICU with a skull fracture. He had been climbing up to a loft in his home when he fell backward off the ladder. The child lost consciousness and his father transported him to the ED. By the time the child arrived in the ED, he had regained consciousness and was alert and active. But he had a significant skull fracture and was thus admitted to the PICU for observation.

In the process of taking a history, the resident discovered that the child had not seen a doctor or received any immunizations since birth. Although child abuse had been considered, the family's story of the events leading up to the skull fracture was consistent and an abuse investigation was not pursued. But child neglect seemed apparent to the healthcare team in the absence of immunizations and well-child visits.

The child did well overnight and could have been discharged home. However, the team decided to transfer him to another unit while social services interviewed the family in more depth. The parents of the child did not agree with the plan to transfer and requested the necessary forms to discharge the child against medical advice. A new plan was made to contact the Department of Children and Families to have the family officially investigated for child neglect if the family left the hospital. The family was made aware of the plan and they proceeded to walk out of the PICU with the child in their arms after signing all the forms.

***

THE USE OF POWER BY HEALTHCARE PROFESSIONALS

CASE 7: WINDOWS

An advanced practice registered nurse (APRN) who is not my preceptor offers to have me tag along with her to see her next patient. After we enter the room, introductions are made and she proceeds with her assessment of the patient. In the course of the assessment, the APRN inquires as to the patient's line of work. The patient says that he is a window installer. The APRN brightens and says, "Oh, how wonderful. I'm having a house built right now. Can I have your card?" As he hands the card to her, she says to me, "You should take one too." The patient hands a card to me as well and says to the APRN, "Well, I'm sure your contractor already has a window company lined up." The APRN quips, "Oh, well, that doesn't matter because I know you will give me the best deal, right? So, I'll have the contractor call you." I am infinitely uncomfortable with what I have just witnessed and am too stunned to determine what it is that I should do, if anything.

CASE 8: Dr. L

A 5-year-old boy, "A," has disclosed anal penetration by his biological father. Dr. L and I were going to take a sexual abuse history from A's mother. Dr. L begins the interview by introducing himself as "Dr. L" and me as "Ms. B," a nurse practitioner student. And he proceeds to call A's mother by her first name. This seemed to label both me and Dr. L as the "professionals" or "the ones in charge," allowing us to dictate the tone and tempo of the visit.

After Dr. L described the purpose of the visit he asked A's mother to describe why she had brought her son to the clinic today. A's mother began to describe the circumstances that led up to the visit. She launched into an hour-long soliloquy about A's story. At this point in the visit, the power dynamic seemed to change. A's mother had all the power in the room. Neither Dr. L nor I could say or do anything while she told her story. It felt as though our only role was to be active listeners.

Usually, I feel in control of visits and that I have the ability to set limits as to the direction of the history. In this situation the control was gone because I was trying to make the visit as nonthreatening as possible and I did not have a time frame in which the visit had to be completed. It felt as though both Dr. L and I needed to "take a back seat" to A's mother until she finished her story in her own words and time.

CASE 9: PALLIATIVE CARE

On the second day of my clinical rotation on the Palliative Care Team I observed the interaction between the attending physician and a patient. The physician entered the room with me and a medical intern and immediately introduced herself to the patient and the patient's daughter. She explained that she was a physician at the hospital and had been asked by Dr. X to come by to see how Louise (the patient) was doing and to see if she could help with her pain.

I witnessed a process of gentle questioning and the slow determination that the patient was getting ready to die and wanted to be relieved of her pain. The Palliative Care Team is only called to see patients with uncontrolled symptoms and/or to discuss end-of-life preparations. Since the team usually does not have an established relationship with the patient, this could be a potential area of conflict. How we enter a room and begin discussion is key. Ultimately, we are strangers, the "bearers of bad news." It is amazing how close we can become to a patient and family after just a few interactions because of the depth and nature of these interactions. This team has an advantage in that there are very few time constraints. We could spend a few minutes or an hour with one patient, whatever it takes.

***

THE HEALTH PROFESSIONAL AS PATIENT OR FAMILY MEMBER

CASE 10: Dr. V

Dr. V's and my goals were similarly oriented around two patients: mother (me) and baby (my unborn child). My objective was to experience labor, a vaginal delivery, and to have a healthy baby. Unlike Dr. V, I took my health for granted and was more focused on the experience.

In fact I did not have the experience I longed for. I ended up with an induction and, ultimately, a c-section. Dr. V is accountable for the outcome of delivery and is legally responsible to perform within practice guidelines. He balanced these requirements along with my goals while not compromising standards of care. His extensive training and education provide him with enormous power over his patients.

Dr. V's working style is to include the patient in decisions whenever possible, or at a minimum provide the patient with the information to understand why certain decisions are being made. Throughout this experience he managed to make it feel like I was a working partner in the decision making. If he was "leading me," he did so without making it feel like manipulation, even in hindsight.

For example, on day 2 postpartum I asked Dr. V if he had known all along that my baby was positioned occiput posterior, even though he didn't share this information with me. He said, "Yes, I knew on exam and just kept charting 'OP,' 'OP,' 'OP.' But you were doing everything possible that would have turned her. That's why we had you changing positions. You were doing everything right."

Dr. V used his professional judgment and chose not to volunteer this information while I was laboring. In retrospect, this information most likely would not have empowered me but would have frustrated me. At the delivery of Olivia Clare, I heard Dr. V say, "Face is up ... big shoulders ... the head's not even molded." To me this information meant we made the right decision. She was OP, we probably avoided a shoulder dystocia, and her head was not even engaged. She was also 9 pounds, 6 ounces!

CASE 11: Dr. P

My mother had been seeing Dr. P for years. As our family doctor, he had seen all of us. He was always a friendly, calm man; the kind of doctor you felt you could rely on. I did realize that my last visit with him was more than 15 years ago and he was white-haired even then. Even in recent years, after word of his multiple divorces and progressively younger wives spread throughout our small town and made me question his personal values, my trust didn't waver in his medical expertise.

Then, my mother got sick. My mother was diagnosed with hypertension. I was away and involved in my own life, but as time passed and I visited home I realized that her kitchen counter had become a pharmacopoeia. She had gained weight and I knew the association between weight gain and hypertension. I assumed that Dr. P was on top of this but that my mother was resisting advice.

As time passed she would talk of being taken on and off various medications and the stress this caused her because of her mediocre insurance coverage. At her last physical, Dr. P was dissatisfied with her BP and doubled one of her medications. But he didn't schedule a follow-up appointment.

A week later my mom telephoned to say that she had been in the ER. She had passed out in the kitchen and, with no one to help her, had driven herself to the hospital. From this moment, I knew that Dr. P was no longer at the top of his game. I advised my mother to change doctors, but she didn't know how to do this. To whom would she go? How could she leave the practice without hurting Dr. P's feelings?

It took one year and two more trips to the ER before my mother got up the courage to ask to be switched to another, younger, doctor in the practice. Much to my surprise, my mom was told "no." Dr. P planned to retire in 8 months and the practice wanted to "honor him" by not switching any of his patients until his retirement was official!

CASE 12: STUDENT AS PATIENT 1

About 5 years ago, I was placed in a situation where I felt powerless as a patient. It is not until now that I fully recognize how little power I gave myself and how much power I afforded the practitioner who was diagnosing and treating me.

I was discovered to have a low platelet count during a routine physical. My primary care physician referred me to a hematologist-oncologist. Upon arriving to my appointment I was escorted to the lab for repeat blood work and asked to wait in a room where the doctor was to see me. I waited nearly a half hour for the doctor, who was to spend 5 minutes of interrupted time with me. He was impersonal, blunt, and seemed to be rushed. I felt as if I were putting him out. During the 5-minute visit, he informed me that I needed to schedule a bone marrow biopsy with no explanation about how it related to the diagnostic process.

On the day of the biopsy I was accompanied by my fiancé, but he was not allowed to remain in the room with me during the procedure. The doctor briskly entered the room and began the procedure. I was not given any options in terms of anesthesia and was injected with a local anesthetic that did not touch the pain I experienced. I was unable to keep my composure and began to cry at which point the doctor responded in an irritable manner that he would never do another biopsy on a young person! Although I was lucky enough to be diagnosed with idiopathic thrombocytopenic purpura and not a more pathological disease, this was an experience that I will never forget.

CASE 13: STUDENT AS PATIENT 2

For the past 6 months I have been undergoing medical and dental treatment for temporomandibular joint (TMJ) dysfunction. My dentist decided to refer me to a specialist after unsuccessfully attempting to manage the disorder. The specialist immediately intimidated me. He never asked me what I did or what I know about my problem. He talked down to me. He gave me a diagnosis and how he planned to treat it. He didn't consult me, ask how I felt about, or if I understood the treatment. After leaving his office I felt confused. I didn't trust the specialist. However, because I trust my dentist and have a great relationship with him, and because he trusts this specialist, I went along with the treatment.

Interprofessional Relationships

Stories in this category fell into three clusters: doctor–nurse, nurse to nurse, and nurse to ancillary workers. Doctor–nurse stories are legion and more often than not negative, depicting the nurse as the victim of the doctor's demeaning outbursts or poor management decisions. The power dynamics between nurses are different and often relate to the distribution of resources or differences of opinion about management plans. The power dynamics between nurses and ancillary personnel are influenced by reporting and supervisory relationships and may also be related to ethnic, racial, and socioeconomic differences.

CASE STUDIES

CASE 1: Ms. KS

Imagine a busy Sunday morning on a full unit. I was called to rounds, but no sooner had I sat down when a man wearing jeans, a button-down shirt, and no identification badge interrupted rounds. He seemed agitated and questioned the pediatric housestaff about whether they had changed diet orders for a certain patient—KS. They denied having done so.

Upon hearing the patient's name, I realized she was a new patient of mine. She had recently undergone a spinal fusion and was being followed by orthopaedic surgery. In a frustrated tone, the man stated that though the patient had been ordered a full liquid diet, there was a tray of food in her room. Though this person had not yet interacted with me, he already exerted power over me. I didn't know his name or exact position, but I guessed he was part of the orthopaedic team.

Because he was visibly unhappy about the care being given to one of his patients, I feared that, as her nurse, I would soon be on the receiving end of his anger. I assumed he must be an attending because of the way he was dressed. No resident would dare wear such casual clothes and fail to display an ID. Thus, I was even more intimidated.

I excused myself from rounds, although it was important that I stay, and approached him and introduced myself as KS's nurse. He began to reprimand me for the tray. I knew that I had given the correct order for a full liquid tray but nevertheless felt responsible for the error and apologized to him. He then proceeded to express his general dissatisfaction with the nursing staff and stated that this type of error "always happens on this unit." And he reprimanded me for the inability to follow orders. Indeed, he ignored my apology and continued to yell at me from the other end of the corridor.

As it turned out, the tray contained milk, cream of wheat, and scrambled eggs, all of which, according to Dietary Services, are part of a full liquid diet. The story goes on, resulting in an eventual letter of apology from the doctor, but not until the nurse manager got in touch with the chair of his department.

Were I able to relive this experience, I would have told him that I was aware of the diet order and probably, in his presence, would have looked up what constitutes a full liquid diet. I mentioned to the charge nurse how angry I was about the interaction to which she replied, "Well, get used to it. You're a nurse."

CASE 2: Miss N

I was a traveling pediatric intensive care nurse at the time that this incident happened. I had been a traveler at this facility for about 4 months, but it was only my second traveling assignment, so I still felt fairly inexperienced. I was the only traveler in the pediatric intensive care unit at the time. Although an outsider, I knew and felt close to the staff and felt like the nurses in the PICU and on the infant and toddler unit knew and respected me as a nurse.

I arrived at work for the night shift and learned that I had been floated to the adolescent unit—where I had not previously worked or been oriented. I started the night feeling powerless. One of the patients assigned to me was a young teenage girl with spina bifida. N had been admitted for an elective G-tube placement due to poor weight gain. When I arrived, the attending physician was explaining to her that she would be going home in the morning.

My night went along like any other until I visited N's room to take her vital signs. They were all out of the normal range! Her pulses were weak and thready, she had tachycardia, her blood pressure was low, and her temperature was low. I knew something wasn't right, but I wasn't sure what it was. I called the senior resident to voice my concerns. He told me he would be up to see her when he had a chance.

By 1:00 a.m. the doctor had still not come, and N's vital signs had not changed. I paged him again, but he did not respond. I paged a third time and told him my concerns. He agreed to come see her and arrived on the floor sometime after 1:30 a.m. He ordered a series of laboratory tests for the morning. I told him I thought we should do something now instead of waiting because she did not look good. His response was that she wasn't complaining, was alert and oriented. I didn't know this resident and was already feeling out of sorts because I didn't know the unit.

By 4:00 a.m. N appeared more anxious and her vital signs were still off. I called the physician several times and he continued to brush me off. I decided to call the attending and the charge nurse from the PICU to come see the girl. By this time she was clearly decompensating. She was taken to the PICU and intubated. I assumed I would be assigned to care for her in the morning.

When I arrived, the charge nurse pulled me aside and told me that N had been taken to surgery because of fluid in the peritoneal cavity and she had died during the operation. I will always wonder if I had just insisted on a KUB (kidney, ureter, and bladder X-ray) from the start or went over the resident's head and called the attending sooner if the outcome would have been very different.

CASE 3: CHARGE NURSE

A total of three registered nurses, including me, were working second shift. One was from the float pool with no oncology experience and would not be assigned care for any patient who was to receive chemotherapy during our shift or anyone recovering from a bone marrow transplant. There were two patients status post bone marrow transplant and four scheduled to receive chemo during the shift. An RN from the first shift with oncology training was willing to work overtime, but the nursing supervisor would not authorize it nor would she allow us to call any of the other oncology nurses because she felt three nurses were adequate to cover the shift. I was casual status and could not take "charge." The float nurse could not take charge either. So, by default the charge nurse was predetermined and she was not happy about it. The float nurse was assigned 7 patients; I was assigned 7 patients; and the charge nurse took 4 patients. The unit norm was for the charge nurse to take one less patient, so I asked her why I had been assigned 7 and she had only taken 4. Her response was that one of my patients was terminal and would likely die before the shift was over and that the patient had several family members in the room who could provide any physical care the patient needed. I attempted to argue that a dying patient actually required more care, but after a short power struggle I was unable to influence her decision and my assignment did not change.

CASE 4: Ms. EA

There is one particular environmental associate (EA), an African American woman, who exerts a great deal of power over nurses and unit management by passive-aggressive and aggressive behavior. On a daily basis she shirks her work, chooses not to do certain tasks, and spends a lot of time on the phone or Internet doing personal business. She knows from experience that because there is a dearth of EAs in the hospital and because she is a person of color and willing to cry "bigotry and prejudice" that no one, including the unit manager, is willing to reprimand her for infractions. Thus, every day our unit is understocked, linen is missing, the kitchen is unwashed, floors go dirty, and discharged patients wait unconscionable amounts of time to be transported. When the charge nurse asks her politely to clean a room or transport a patient, she will respond at her own speed with some flip answer to show that she may or may not do the task and it will be at her own pleasure.... The unit manager is not willing to use her organizational power to require compliance, and people are in general uncomfortable with confrontation, which the EA is happy to exercise. Power can be assigned, but if the person in possession of the power does not use it, she may lose it.

Student–Faculty Relationships

Clearly, there are power dynamics in all academic relationships. The professor holds the power to evaluate and grade students. Many of the courses students take are required for graduation and/or certification and licensure. Students have the capacity to give or withhold full participation in a course, thus affecting overall quality of the teaching-learning experience. The student–faculty relationship in the clinical setting is a special instance in which it is expected that the faculty will model effective clinical relationships. Power dynamics in the clinical setting are heightened because of the increased vulnerability of patients and students. The following examples illustrate clinical management disagreements between student and preceptor, positive clinical role modeling by a faculty member, differences in practice cultures, and communication problems between students in a specialty and the administration. Taken together they suggest that students (perhaps like patients) are neither as powerless as they feel nor are they always able to effect immediate change.

CASE STUDIES

CASE 1: JAN

Jan, a 64-year-old woman, is seeing me for a follow-up visit. Her problem list on the inside cover of her chart shows type 1 diabetes, cardiovascular disease, diabetic neuropathy, nephropathy, depression, hypertension, chronic low back pain, and well adult care (an oxymoron?). Everything looks good but her finger stick blood sugar, which is 468.

We discuss her diabetes regimen. She's on NPH (a type of insulin) twice a day and rarely checks her sugar at home. She isn't sure why she doesn't test her sugar and admits to forgetting her insulin about three to four times a week. She eats irregularly, sometimes only once a day, and follows no diet plan. She lives alone, does not work, and has no form of physical activity.

I do a quick exam, but what I really want to do is get her blood sugar down to a safer level. Throughout the visit, all I can think of is insulin, this woman needs insulin. I leave the room to discuss the visit with my preceptor. I indicate that I think I should give Jan some regular or Humalog in the office—I am very confident of this plan.

To my surprise, my preceptor disagrees, "Jan's blood sugar is well controlled when she takes her insulin. When she doesn't take it, it's not. Giving her insulin here in the office is only going to be a solution for the immediate problem. We're going to send her home and she won't take her medication again and then we're back to square one. Do what you want, but we can't help her if she doesn't do what she is supposed to do."

From where did my instructor's frustrations regarding Jan's compliance come? Since, for the most part, I respect my instructor's clinical decision making and patient–provider interactions, I have to assume that Jan has more power in this situation than I think. Jan does have the power to control the symptoms of this chronic illness and "own" an aspect of her health. Despite the clinic's best efforts, she does not do so.

So, here I am, a student. In front of me sit a patient feeling powerless, who is labeled with a powerful illness, and a clinical instructor, who has the power to judge Jan, her diagnosis, me, and all of our futures. However, I do remember my instructor saying, "Do what you want," so I do. I give Jan 26 units of regular insulin, which she administers herself. Her blood sugar declines and she goes on her way. She made an appointment to see me in 2 weeks. I am looking forward to building a relationship with her and helping her regain some control over her own health care.

CASE 2: PRECEPTOR

It was my first day as a student at my clinical site. There was a multiparous woman in labor to whom I was assigned. Upon arrival to the patient's room, I introduced myself and reviewed her medical records and the progress of her labor. The woman was coping well and progressing, and the fetal heart rate looked great. I discussed the situation with my preceptor (who was a provider at the clinical site), and we both agreed that we anticipated a vaginal delivery of a baby with an estimated fetal weight of 7.5 pounds, smaller than any of the woman's previous babies.

After 1 hour, the woman was 10 cm dilated and pushing effectively. I gowned and gloved for the birth. My preceptor, standing behind me, asked if I had ever cut an episiotomy. I said no. She said, "You are going to cut one now." I asked why an episiotomy was indicated, and the preceptor said, "Because you have to learn how to do it." I hesitated because I was very reluctant to perform what I saw as an unnecessary procedure just for a learning experience.

The preceptor noticed my hesitation, so she picked up the scissors and without explaining to the woman what was happening, cut an episiotomy, never asking the woman for her permission or explaining the procedure to her. The baby was born vigorous and healthy.

Afterward, I inquired why my preceptor had cut the episiotomy when it wasn't indicated. Her response was she "thought I needed to learn how to do it and it makes babies come out faster, which is an issue at the hospital with a busy labor floor and patients always waiting in the wings." I later learned that the record indicated the patient had asked not to have an episiotomy and, to this date, I wonder whether she is even aware what occurred during the delivery.

CASE 3: THE MIDWIFE

We are in a labor and delivery unit in a rural, government hospital in South Africa. It is 110 degrees Fahrenheit, there is no breeze, and there are very few windows in the unit. A 17-year-old girl is laboring with her first baby. She is fully dilated and can now begin pushing. She is tired and scared, having been laboring alone all day in the hospital lobby, and is now being cared for by me (nurse-midwifery student)—a white woman who does not speak her language. A South African midwife comes into the room and speaks to the patient. The midwife speaks English fluently, but does not talk to me directly until I ask her what she has said to the patient. She states she has explained to the patient that she can start pushing.

An hour passes. I have been trying to reassure and encourage the young woman using any available hospital staff to interpret for me. I use the little Zulu I know to communicate otherwise. I call her by name frequently. She is making progress. The South African midwife comes into the room several times and yells at the patient in Zulu. My preceptor, whom I accompanied on this trip, is busy in another room but checks on me as much as possible. The South African midwife, now available to "help" as she says, returns to the room. She puts on sterile gloves, starts yelling at the patient loudly, and begins to roughly slap the patient across the face and on the chest. She uses these same gloves to conduct a vaginal exam to examine the station of the baby. All along the midwife does not speak to me.

I am short. The patient has a small build, but that seems irrelevant as she is already in the most vulnerable position of the three of us. What do I say? I feel paralyzed, but I need to help my patient. I need my teacher—she'll help me. I peek out from behind the curtain to the larger room. My teacher sees me and comes in. My teacher tells the midwife that she will stay with me for the rest of the delivery; she suggests that the midwife "take a break from this hard work." The midwife leaves the room. My teacher and I help this patient deliver her baby. We cannot speak her language, but we use our compassion to communicate our concern for her. My teacher helped the patient to a better outcome and helped the South African midwife save face—an important intervention since we depend on the South African midwife for our experience.

CASE 4: ADMINISTRATION

A series of events within a specialty program led to this final story about faculty, students, and administrators. We pick up the story as the students attempt to diagnose and resolve the problems. During an informal discussion after class, several students began to express concern to each other about incidents that had occurred within the program. It became clear that these were not simply a random collection of individual incidents but rather a significant problem with communication, organization, and timeliness within the program.

The conversation revealed that many students had been attempting resolution of various problems through the specialty director's office with little or no response. It was decided that the students should meet as a group, identify their concerns, and request a meeting with the associate dean. The students' goals were to clarify the issues, increase their collective power, provide a "neutral buffer" between themselves and the specialty director, and attempt to address the problems while following proper protocol.

Timeliness was an issue because the semester was rapidly coming to a close. It took the associate dean a total of 4 weeks to set up a meeting with the students and the director. The students submitted a list of their concerns in advance. The meeting seemed tense for all involved, but the students left feeling cautiously optimistic that their concerns had been heard and would be addressed.

Unfortunately, all did not go as planned. When the next semester began it became apparent that much remained unchanged and the communication problems persisted—in fact, they had become more adversarial. The students met again and, despite some frustration and wariness, agreed to request a group meeting with the dean. A meeting was scheduled, and the students once again submitted a list of concerns a week ahead of time. With only one day's notice, the dean canceled the meeting because of a scheduling conflict and the students were encouraged to go back to the associate dean to discuss further problems.

The students believed that despite their attempts to address problems in a direct and assertive manner, they were being given the message that their concerns didn't warrant the attention of the administration—the very people upon whom they depended to make any changes.

While the students were deciding what to do next, the associate dean scheduled another meeting with all parties involved. The students went to the meeting resolved to be respectful but more assertive. They added to their list of concerns the fact that the organization as a whole seemed unresponsive and lacking in accountability. The administration seemed appropriately sobered by both the magnitude and the longstanding nature of the problems and made a commitment to resolve the issues. The students requested a follow-up meeting midway through the semester to review progress.

Although it had been difficult, time-consuming, and uncomfortable, the students felt they had conveyed the message that their concerns were legitimate and could significantly affect the future reputation of the program. Although they would have preferred not to experience any of the conflicts, the situation ultimately provided a significant learning experience about the value of collective power in problem solving as well as the significance of assertiveness, perseverance, and respect for others' opinions and experiences.

Systems Relationships

Systems relationships are characterized as interactions and transactions that take place at the administrative level or within an organization as a whole. Stories in this category represented four clusters: power dynamics at the administrative or management level, those emanating from organizational culture, those resulting from interorganizational transactions, and those that emerge from systems-wide policies. These issues are often comingled in a single story but represent different types of power dynamics.

CASE STUDIES

CASE 1: THE PHYSICIAN

This case involves the male MD who is the director of the division. He has had many years of practice in his specialty and as an administrator and is a charismatic and visionary leader. He has a national research reputation. But he is not a flexible or open negotiator. The case also involves a female director of nursing for the division. She is intelligent, articulate, and visionary and is known to be an excellent negotiator who is well attuned to political dynamics.

The unit has a vacancy in a nurse manager position. The unit is well known as an excellent place to work with high scores for patient satisfaction and staff retention. Historically, the selection process for nurse managers does not involve physicians in the interview or consultation process. The director of nursing proceeded with interviews. However, the MD director referred an outside candidate of his choice. In the end, the director of nursing selected an inside candidate.

A few weeks later the MD director circulated an email to a large number of administrators and clinicians in the institution expressing his objections to the selection process and to the candidate who was selected. In the meantime, the candidate had already begun the process of transition to the position. Discussion and debate ensued that resulted in a change in process going forward. Henceforth, physicians would be involved in the selection of nurse managers.

CASE 2: THE PHARMACY

The lights were out. The door was locked. No one was there, and it was after 9:00 a.m. on a brisk Wednesday morning. There were several confused looks on people's faces. They knocked on the door. They knocked louder. No one came to the door. The door stayed locked. The lights stayed off. They went upstairs to the clinic, a few people at a time. They demanded to know why the pharmacy was closed today. The clinicians looked at one another. Their looks of confusion betrayed the patients. No one knew why the pharmacy was closed. They all began muttering to one another. They were all frustrated and angry. "Typical about the way things go in this clinic" was a comment heard by all. Yesterday at 5:00 p.m. the pharmacy closed for the night. The pharmacist turned off the lights and said goodbye for the last time. At 6:00 p.m., after many of the clinicians had left for the evening, the administration announced that the pharmacy was severing its relationship with the clinic because the clinic had been unable to pay a $95,000 past-due bill.

CASE 3: THE PEDIATRICIAN

I have clinical rotation assignments at two different sites. One is a private practice in an affluent part of the state and my preceptor is a pediatrician who had been in practice for 30 years. The other is at a military base where I was precepted by a young physician only 2 years out of a residency program and by a nurse practitioner who had 20 years of experience.

At first, both sites were similar—I was required to "shadow" my preceptors, not engaging in much hands-on practice. By the third week at the military base, my preceptors began to allow me some autonomy, at first remaining in the room while I conducted an exam and then, once comfortable with my skill level, leaving me to conduct the history alone, then the physical exam, etc. The philosophy at the base was watch a procedure, do a procedure, teach a procedure. By the end of the term I had performed colposcopy with MD supervision, surgically removed nevi and skin tags, and performed wart removals.

Meanwhile back at the private practice I was still shadowing the pediatrician, at times being allowed to examine a patient, but never without the physician in the room. The physician always repeated the exam after me, and I was not allowed to chart in the patient record. As I spend more time in private practice I've noticed that many patients ask almost immediately if the physician will be seeing them when the nurse practitioner is finished—as if they have no confidence in the NP. In addition, it seems that MDs in private practice undermine the nurse practitioner profession as a whole by requiring unreasonable levels of physician supervision not required under the Nurse Practice Act.

CASE 4: THE MILITARY

As the weeks have passed and the semester has progressed, what I perceived as hostility on my first day at the Naval Base has diminished. I think back on that day often, and although my family and friends laugh at the tale I tell, there is something about it that continues to feel unsettling. When I drove home on the evening of my first day at the base, I tried to make sense of the experience, to understand why I felt so disrespected and confined. From obtaining a pass and providing information for an FBI security check, to feeling as if my clothes were looked upon as not well enough starched, to the comment from a medical assistant who laughed at my clogs and commented "nice shoes" with a smirk, to the corpsmen who called me Ma'am, to the physician who didn't even acknowledge my presence—there was a laundry list of ways that power made its mark on my day.

I have come to understand that in the military, the culture of respect is one of hierarchy. I know this from stories my father tells of being in the Navy during the Korean War. The conflict I experienced on my first day was about respect and power. Rank is recognized and there are rules about who can socialize with whom. In the broader context, I like to think that the rigidity and power that I experienced on the first day was a cultural difference. Once I became more accustomed to the atmosphere of a military setting, more comfortable in my sense of place there, I began to feel that it wasn't something personal. Order and power are essentially what the military is all about.

CASE 5: THE CRISIS INTERVENTION UNIT

This scenario took place in the emergency department of a large, urban teaching hospital. The key players were representatives of the psychiatric area of the ED (the Crisis Intervention Unit—CIU) and the larger medical area of the ED. There was a triad of new clinical service managers, two from the adult ED and one from the pediatric ED, but each of these managers had assumed the administrative position after a long career as a medical ED nurse. None had worked in psychiatry.

On the day of the event, both the psych and medical EDs were percolating with activity. The CIU had been at capacity for several days. It is designed as an area to evaluate patients with acute mental illness and to create a suitable disposition plan. On this particular day we remained over capacity and, by protocol, were not taking more patients who had been triaged on the medical side.

Occasionally, the triage nurse from medical would arrive unannounced, be buzzed in, and walk through the unit glancing around with an angry demeanor as if checking on the validity of our report that we were still closed to new admissions. At another point the triage nurse escorted a very psychotic patient onto the unit, failing to give us a report, and on her way out muttered within earshot of the patient and others "better you than me."

Finally, at the end of the shift the back door opened and in walked security, the triage nurse, and a new patient. The triage nurse declared that "Dr. M [the medical ER attending] said that we could bring this patient back since he's medically cleared and has been waiting over there since 3 a.m. last night." Moments later, Dr. M arrived in the CIU looking irritable, entered the nurse's station, and said, "Look, I can't have these people just hanging around my ER. Just get on the phone and book this guy a bed!"

CASE 6: MEDICAID

A 51-year-old woman with Medicaid came to our office for follow-up after an ER visit. She had fallen down stairs and suffered from knee pain. In the ER, X-rays were taken that revealed no fractures. According to the patient, she had been instructed to go home, rest, and take over-the-counter pain relief as needed. At follow-up she believed her condition had worsened and reported bilateral knee pain including sharp pain that radiated from her right hip to her right knee. After a thorough exam we decided she needed a brace, to continue RICE, and to avoid walking when possible. We ordered an MRI and referred her to orthopaedics for further evaluation. The MRI showed fractures of the tibia and fibula as well as a meniscal tear of the right knee. Because she was on Medicaid no orthopedist would agree to see her. We sent her back to the ER (of a different hospital) so that the orthopedist on call would have to see her and evaluate her injuries. She was seen by a resident, given a walker, and told to make an appointment with an orthopedist. She was finally able to get an appointment at the orthopaedic clinic based at the hospital and was prescribed physical therapy.

CASE 7: THE INSURANCE COMPANY

The consulting physician, my preceptor, and I all agreed that Mrs. B needed a CT scan; her insurance company did not. The medical assistant fought with the insurance company on the phone for over half an hour and she was unable to get authorization. Next, my preceptor called. She spoke with a different person, explaining Mrs. B's history and why we felt the CT scan was necessary. The insurance company continued to deny authorization. During this time, Mrs. B was sitting in the waiting room, probably nervous and scared. Next, the consulting physician called the insurance company. Authorization was still denied. Now, it was 4 p.m. on a Friday. The consulting physician made the decision to send Mrs. B for the CT without authorization. We told her to go get it done and we would get authorization later. The following week, we learned that the CT scan showed a mass and subsequently Mrs. B was diagnosed with lung cancer. Her insurance company gave authorization after learning the results.

As all of these stories illustrate, power is a relational concept. It is a dynamic concept that is worked out in relationship to others. People are always measuring self-power in relation to others. Power applies to the dyad as well as to organizations and interprofessional relations. One has personal power, relationship power, and environmental power. All of these concepts are relevant to the healthcare relationship. The most important idea is that, absent a relational construct, power cannot be apprehended or understood. Yet power is what frames healthcare relationships and transactions.

DISCUSSION QUESTIONS

1. How would you explain the overwhelming emphasis in the stories on the negative aspects of power?

2. The idea of patients as victims or as powerless comes up a lot. In fact, the idea of nurses as victims or powerless comes up almost as much. Are there ways to reframe the power dynamics in clinical encounters to avoid victimization?

3. Where does empowerment fit in the conceptualization of power in healthcare relationships? Is empowerment always the right goal?

4. In what ways do theoretical, ethical, and practical understandings of power dynamics in healthcare relationships and transactions influence how we legislate, regulate, organize, and implement healthcare services for patients?

5. Do these stories capture the universe of important power dynamics in health care or can you think of other examples that were not mentioned?

References

Alcabes, P., & Williams, A. (2002). Human rights and the ethic of care: A framework for health research and practice. *Yale Journal of Health, Policy, Law, and Ethics, 2*(2), 229–254.

Cassell, E. J. (1991). *The nature of suffering.* New York, NY: Oxford University Press.

Fins, J. J. (1999). Commentary: From contract to covenant in advance care planning. *Journal of Law, Medicine and Ethics, 27*(1), 46–51.

Fins, J. J., Miller, F. G., & Bacchetta, M. D. (1998). Clinical pragmatism: Bridging theory and practice. *Kennedy Institute of Ethics Journal, 8*(1), 37–42.

Fins, J. J., & Solomon, M. Z. (2001). Communication in intensive care settings: The challenge of futility disputes. *Critical Care Medicine, 29*(2), N10–N15.

Freire, P. (1972). *Pedagogy of the oppressed* (M. Bergman Ramos, Trans.). New York, NY: Herder and Herder.

Grossman, S., & Valiga, T. (2005). *The new leadership challenge: Creating the future of nursing.* Philadelphia, PA: F. A. Davis.

Henderson, S., & Fins, J. J. (1998). Resuscitation in hospice. *Hastings Center Report, 28*(6), 20–22.

Hill, L. (1995). *Power and influence.* Cambridge, MA: Harvard Business School Publishing.

Levi, B. H. (1999). *Respecting patient autonomy.* Chicago: University of Illinois Press.

Tomey, A. (2000). *Guide to nursing management and leadership* (6th ed.). St. Louis, MO: Mosby.

Yoder, S. D. (2002). Individual responsibility for health: Decision, not discovery. *Hastings Center Report, 32*(2), 22–23.

Index

Note: *Boxes, figures, and tables are indicated by b, f, and t following page numbers.*